YOGA FOR CHILDREN

A guide for parents to incorporate 5 "S" s of yoga to Improve self-control, discipline, self-esteem, Concentration, Attention Span and Memory in their children's lives

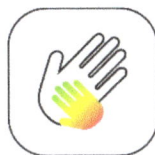

Newbee Publication

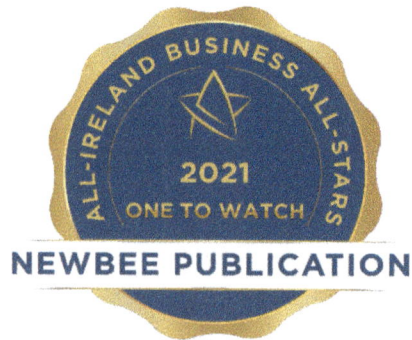

ALL-IRELAND BUSINESS ALL-STARS

2021
ONE TO WATCH

NEWBEE PUBLICATION

Table of Contents

INTRODUCTION

Yoga for children and teenagers is becoming increasingly popular worldwide with the growing popularity of yoga among all adults. Adults understand how beneficial Yoga practice for children in their lives.

Children are like a seed; they need a nurturing environment to grow. If we give a nurturing environment to seed, it becomes a beautiful and big tree. Children also need a nurturing environment, and they adapt everything from that environment. As a parent, our role is to provide a nurturing and safe environment to them, and we can watch and feel proud of how they expand their branches to all areas of life.

In the current environment, you probably have observed that kids' physical activities have tremendously reduced. They sit in classrooms for the whole day in schools. Children are badly affected when Covid encountered in different countries. And they are forced to sit in front of computers and mobiles for online classes or assignments. And after a tiring day of online study, they spend on TV and video games whenever time left.

There is no physical activity left for children, and as we all know, children are full of energy. They feel comfort in playing fast-moving games on television to balance their access energy out. The fast-moving games are high energy games. It seems like children are very attentive and focused. But games are continually shifting their focus. They are moving from one area to another to achieve a reward and win the game. It is understood that playing these high moving games develops a habit of shifting focus from one task to another task. At the same time, they are high energy games and filled children with more energy. You can notice behaviour issues arise when they lose the game or turn off their games. They do not know how to channel this extra energy. We need to guide them on how to channelise this energy and use it in the right direction.

Yoga is a discipline that is linked to the development of physical and mental wellbeing. It means "union" in Sanskrit, meaning – the union of body, mind, and spirit. Experts recognised it as ideal for maintaining a relaxed body by channelising extra energy, toning the body, improving concentration, focus and attention span and even fighting deadly diseases.

Children's bodies and minds are readily and easily susceptible to new learning and adapting to new postures. If proper coaching is offered, they will become more organised and improve their confidence and self-esteem.

Most kids are under tremendous stress these days—endless homework, tough competition, relationships with students and peer pressure, etc. To deal with various issues, they must learn how to calm themselves and take the right decision. Children will learn ways to relax and get rid of the tension in their lives with yoga.

Many studies have shown that many kids who practice yoga can focus for more extended periods. It is a reality that many fascinating things will divert their attention. Yoga practice, however, will help kids learn to concentrate their minds more efficiently. Proper breathing, exercise and deep relaxation can be the powerful healing force required in an era in which children acquire disorders and diseases previously unknown in infancy.

The "Yoga Sutra," a 2,000year-old scripted by the Indian sage Patanjali and mentioned yogic philosophy, is a guidebook on how to master the mind, control emotions, and develop spiritually. The Yoga Sutra is one of the oldest texts in existence.

Great yogis have passed this discipline on to their students. Students then open several yoga schools. As the practice extended, it becomes popular and expanded its global scope and popularity.

Yoga is well known for its stances and poses. Still, in India, they were not a core component of yoga's original practices. Fitness was not a primary focus. Instead, practitioners and adherents of the yogic tradition focused on other activities, such as breathing exercises and mental concentration, to expand spiritual capacity.

At the end of the 19th century, the practice started gaining traction in the West. Then, in the 1920s and 1930s, an explosion of interest in postural yoga occurred, first in India and later in the West.

CHAPTER ONE
Yoga for Children

The Yoga for Kids is a cure for growing well physically and emotionally and learning how to socialise in a fun and enjoyable environment.

The practise of yoga helps the little ones be aware of their body and the importance of breathing, develop altruistic behaviour, and learn the importance of respecting others.

How to practice yoga with children:
It is essential to keep in mind that yoga should be introduced as a play and fun activity for the little ones.

It is always ideal to start training your children with yoga early when they are toddlers. Because that is the age of exploration and growth. Parents are supermodels for them. That is why you have noticed that they copy everything their parents do, even how they talk on the telephone, walk and act in different situations. They follow their parents,which is the best time to train them and sit with them in yoga poses to develop a habit. Both parents must sit together to follow the ritual to give a clear message to the little one's exploring brains.

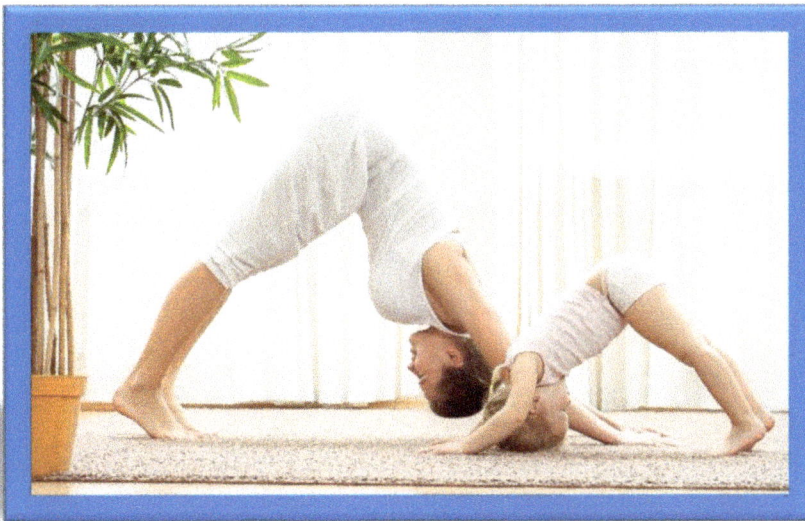

Team or couple games, warm-up exercises, and asanas specially selected for children are suitable for their development phase.

Yoga for children can last from 30 to 40 minutes, depending on the participants' age. Several elements can be introduced to make it enjoyable, like listening to relaxing music, dancing, and singing, storytelling dedicated to fundamental themes such as friendship, respecting others and the environment, and moments dedicated to art and emotions.

The movements in the practice of asanas are always gentle, slow, and guide children's total safety. Each child should have a mat and wear non-slip socks.

Yoga for children must take place in a playful atmosphere and a comfortable and welcoming environment and get the ability to relate to family members. A parent becomes the protagonists of stories to demonstrate the poses to children and small theatrical performances. Towards the end, a moment dedicated to relaxation and short meditation cannot be missed.

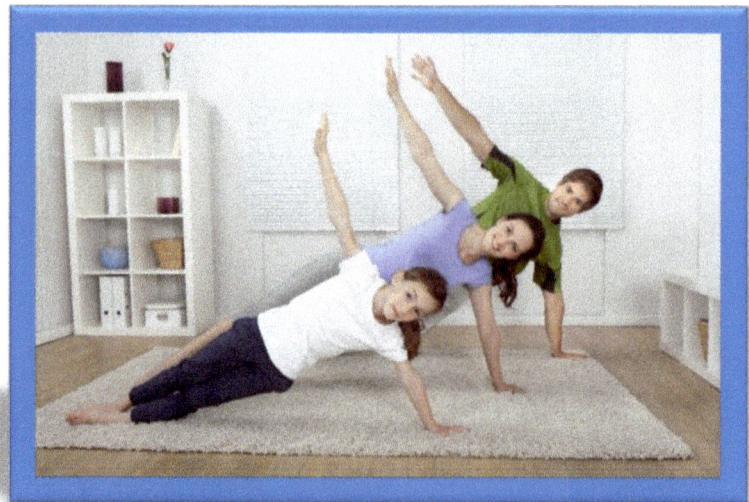

Meditation for Children

As for adults, meditation is a beneficial moment of relaxation for children. Yoga sessions for children can be concluded with a few minutes of meditation or relaxation, with a duration ranging from a couple of minutes to 10-15 minutes.

The Benefits of Yoga for Children

Practicing yoga from an early age can be a source of numerous benefits that should not be underestimated. Let us think about how many hours children dedicate to school and homework while sitting for a long time. They should devote a substantial portion of their time to play and movement, but increasingly this is not the case. Yoga helps restore a healthy balance between commitments, fun, and relaxation in children's days.

The physical results of yoga are improved flexibility, strength, coordination, balance, and awareness of one's body. In addition, it helps you relax and calm down. Thus, children get the best of both worlds: playtime, physical activity, and being in touch with themselves, others, and the world around them. We can thus summarise the main benefits of yoga for children. Practicing yoga from an early age is beneficial for:

- Improve concentration
- Stimulate balance and elasticity.
- Promote freedom of expression.
- Develop awareness of the breath and one's body.
- Devote more time to play as a fundamental tool for growth.
- Improve self-knowledge and socialisation.
- Express emotions and moods in the best possible way.
- Reduce anxiety, stress, and aggression.
- To nourish the rational and emotional intelligence to learn about the world.
- Stimulate learning ability.

A simple yoga routine can negate the overstimulation children experience nowadays. Yoga sculpts young minds and bodies early, providing tools that will enrich and support children to be balanced, creative, and calm individuals with a strong sense of individuality. It enhances self-esteem, concentration, body awareness, and the ability to smoothly deal with life's challenges. Physically, yoga improves coordination, and it has a powerful effect on brain development and brings heightened focus.

1. **It Enhances Physical Flexibility**:

Children are flexible. They can turn their body, twist, and hide in the smallest place where you can never imagine. As they grow, their muscles start to tighten up, and flexibility reduces. However, if children are doing yoga regularly, they stay flexible. Yoga enhances the flexibility of whether a position is done standing, sitting, or resting. Children can challenge specific muscles and achieve maximum flexibility.

2. **It Refines Balance and Coordination:**

Yoga increases balance and coordination in children. Yoga is combined with fine-motor and gross-motor coordination exercises. Certain yoga poses require kids to balance their hands, palms, and legs. These poses strengthen the hands and arm's intrinsic muscles needed for writing, drawing, holding, and picking fine objects and other fine motor tasks. And A strong core and postural muscles needed for gross motor skills such as running, walking, skipping, playground skills, sport, etc.

3. **It Develops Focus and Concentration:**

It is a well-known fact that yoga increases focus and concentration. While doing different poses or sitting in meditation, learning to control breathing, all yogic exercises need focus and attention. With the regular habit of sitting in a yoga pose, you increase focus and concentration. While focusing on the breath and providing oxygen to the brain increase the brain's blood circulation, engagement, and attention.

4. **It Boosts Self-Esteem and Confidence:**

As children grow in yoga, they develop a confident self-image because they slowly start to see the world differently and their perception changes. They stop comparing and complaining as they engage with their inner selves.

5. It Strengthens the Mind-Body Connection:

Yoga is the "union" of body, mind, and soul. Yoga aligns and intensifies connections and advances body and mental ability to perform better.

NPR has a detailed study done by special educators. They introduced an everyday yoga program at a Bronx government-funded school. They found that the program diminished children's violent conduct, social withdrawal, hyperactivity, disagreement.

Kristie Patten Koenig, PhD, a partner educator of word-related treatment at New York University, has driven the examination. She stated that yoga was successful because it appeared to play to children's mental imbalance and decreasing pressure. Yoga helps address children's elevated nervousness and powerless self-esteem parameter.

6. Yoga Improves Memory and Cognitive Functioning

Yoga assists in improving memory and cognitive functioning. Yoga benefits the brain in ways similar to aerobic exercise (1). The study published in the journal Brain Plasticity has shown an improvement in cognitive performance, attention, and memory.

For the study, researchers reviewed 11 studies that looked at the effects of practising yoga on the brain. They found that yoga appears to have a positive effect on key areas "responsible for memory and information processing, as well as emotional regulation" (2)

7. Yoga Improves Social Relationships

Yoga is seen as a solo activity, but doing it with a group or with family members can add social flavour. The use of music, songs, and other fun activities when doing yoga with children creates a positive and engaging environment, boosting their self-esteem, self-confidence, and behaviour. This positive attitude reflects on their relationship with everyone.

8. Yoga Reduces Stress and Anxiety and Improves Sleep:

Adults often think that kids do not have any stress and pressure, but this is not true. They are also dealing with various aspects of life, and they have their own way of reacting and coping. For example, they might be stressed out by their schoolwork, teachers, friends, siblings, and other relationships.
Yoga helps kids to relieve stress and to breathe properly to calm the mind and the nervous system. Yoga releases negative emotions held physically in the body, allowing them to fall asleep faster and stay asleep longer.

9. Yoga Increases Determination and Perseverance:

Practising different yoga poses and succeeding under challenging poses increases the satisfaction of attainment, slowly growing their determination and perseverance to achieve more challenging poses.

10. Yoga Improves Independence and Coping Skills:

Balancing Yoga improves confidence and self-esteem. Yoga fills kids with positive energy, and that energy helps them make independent decisions and cope with different situations.

11. Yoga Improves Mood:

Yoga changes the brain's chemistry. When we practice yoga, activate different chakras. These chakras are responsible for maintaining the seven most important endocrine glands that regulate bodily function by releasing hormones. Endocrine glands play a vital role in wellbeing and happiness. Children can balance their Chakras by practising different poses and elevate mood swings and increase cheerfulness.

12. Yoga supports positive mental prosperity in children:

As children recognise healthy ways of living and love themselves, they can see others' positive characteristics and make focused and calm decisions. They will undoubtedly be optimistic about their abilities.

13. Yoga helps youth to stay in the present and away from addiction:

Yoga has been proven to help calm the nervous system. It relaxes the muscles and mental synapses for times when the addictive nature of a person is triggered. Yoga helps them to identify psychological and physical destructive habits. Many yoga exercises can help youth calm their minds and focus on the present and positive ways to lead life. (4)

Where to Practice Yoga for Children:

 It is essential to set a yoga ritual that includes sitting every day at the same time and at the same place. Make a schedule either morning or evening for a family to sit together and do yoga. It can be started as family time or chat time and slowly introduce breathing. When the habit is forming to take shape, time to start poses. Never force your children; the atmosphere should be calming and fun-filled. Children learn faster if they enjoy the activity.

The room should have an optimum temperature, an open window for fresh air, or it can be done in your back garden in the fresh air under the sun.

Once a ritual is formed, you can change the Yoga place to increase the mindfulness (e.g., living room, sitting in the front garden or back garden, park, open area of your house etc.) depending on weather conditions and location.

CHAPTER TWO
Yoga for Children - Improve Self Control

Self-regulation is an instrument we can provide in our lives that is sometimes ignored and very teachable. Nowadays, children must learn how to control themselves from different negative influences and how to regulate thoughts.

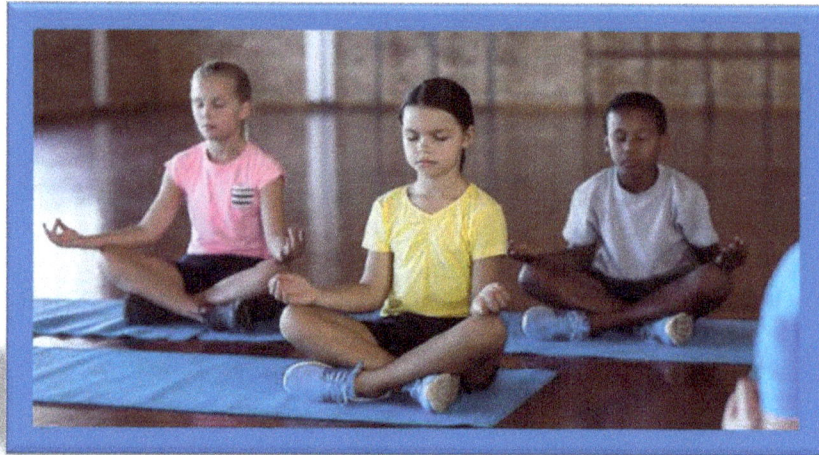

Let us start with a simple self-regulation concept. Wikipedia describes emotional self-regulation as "the ability to respond to the ongoing demands of experience with the range of emotions in a way that is socially tolerable and flexible enough to allow spontaneous reactions." Think about all that is thrown at us daily, and then think about being a child and not having spontaneous reactions as needed. You will start to see why there are tantrums, fights, screaming, attitudes, and hair-pulling.

The goal of self-regulation is to make it possible for our social movement to succeed in the world. To get along with others, turn up for daily rituals, set up and maintain relations, live in a community, we must learn self-regulation skills.

Angela Wilson, a blogger, researcher, and yoga science instructor, explains self-regulation: "Yoga provides both "top-down" tools (i.e., tools that affect the mind) and "bottom-up tools" (tools that affect the body), and it is this synergistic effect that creates the most impact, unique to yoga."

This means that it is imperative to integrate breathing practice. All of this helps the concept of "change the body, change the mind" to take hold. And we need to understand, of course, why these pieces and sections help us self-regulate: when we stop responding, we allow ourselves to choose a better response.

The absence of self-regulation may appear to be both personality-driven and environment-driven. In other words, kids with apparent difficulties in self-regulation because they are vulnerable to it or because they have been subjected to a flawed role model. Nevertheless, experts strongly recommend developing self-regulation skills; parents, educators, and caregivers create a system of encouragement and set a practice time.

I came across this quote recently, and it almost blew my mind: "in its practice, the whole of virtue consists." Marcus Tullius Cicero is attributed to it. Even though it is talking about morality's actions, shift the term to self-regulation from virtue. Or something that you are trying to master because it is the facts. We must practice so that second nature becomes the desired behaviour/skill/ability.

Of course, breathing is an important thing! A decent discussion of breathing and the ability to practice deep belly breaths and shallow bunny breaths should be part of the yoga session.

I take yoga classes in various primary and secondary schools, and I always explain to students that the fastest way to calm ourselves down spontaneously is to concentrate on deep breaths.

Meditation is an enormous self-regulation mechanism. Choose a mantra-like: "I am in control," "Now I am calm." Emphasise repetition's meaning.

Introduce any items you might have for calming down, such as sensory jars, or drawing mandalas, or playing dough, or a cube of Rubik, or bubbles, or puzzles. Google that! A calm-down kit would be a fantastic idea in every home and classroom.

Yoga Poses to Improve self-control:

1. **Tree Pose:**

- Stand erect and tall
- Balance your body on one leg
- Slowly place your one leg on another
- Stay in that position until you are en
- Breath in and slowly raises your hands, and join your palms in the N
- Hold your breath a few second
- Breath out and bring your hands and leg down; repeat with anot
- Repeat 3 times with both legs.

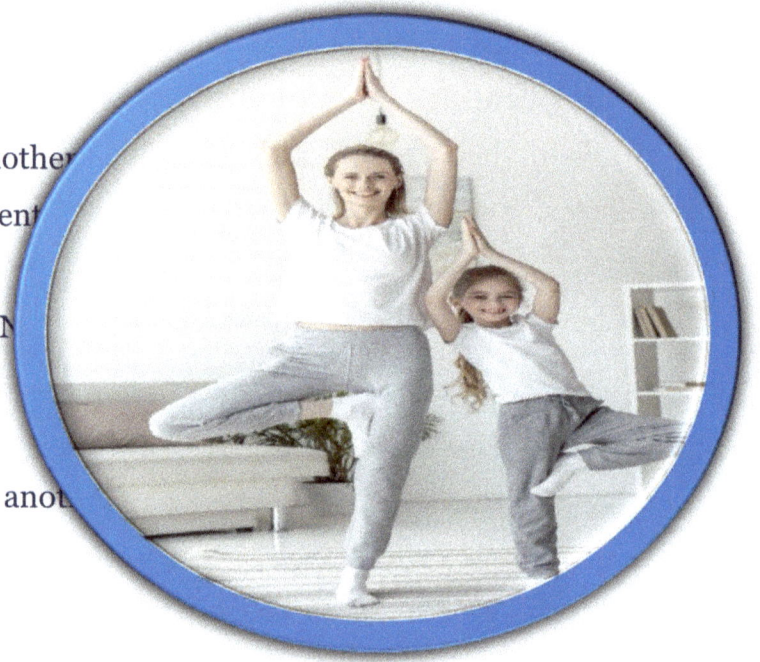

2. Warrior Pose:

- Stand tall with back and neck st
- Move your right leg forward
- Bend your forward leg knee in a
- Stretch your arms in a straight
- Maintain the position for 10 sec
- Repeat 3 times from both legs.

3. Warriors pose:
- Same steps instead of raising ar arms overhead.
- Breath- in and stretch your arm
- Stretch as much as you can; hold your breath and hold the position for 10 seconds.
- Breath out and change legs.
- Repeat steps from both legs 3 times.

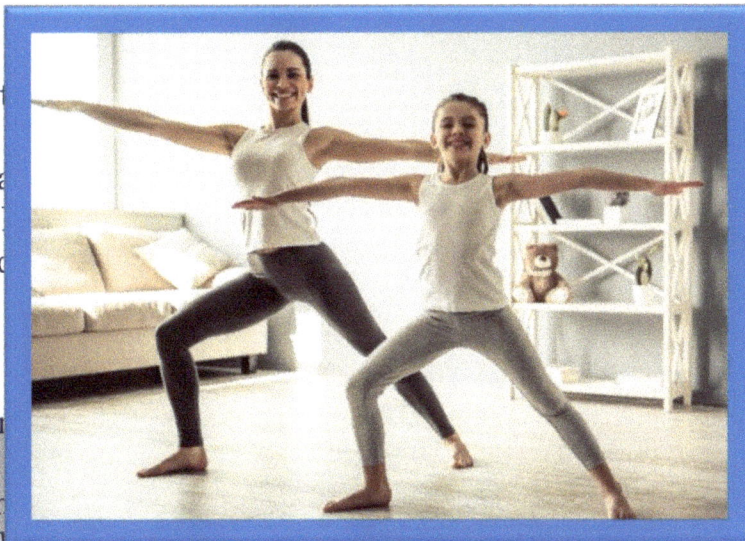

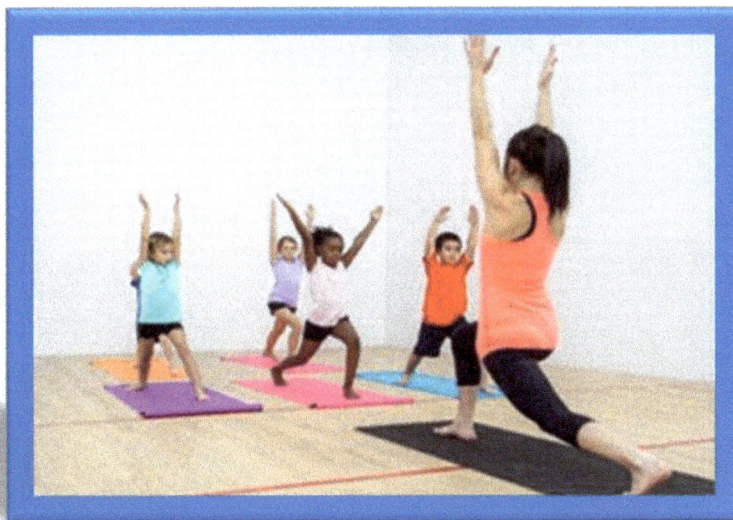

4. Angles pose 1:

- Stand tall and put your legs one or two steps apart from ea... your flexibility)
- Put your left hand close to your left ear and your right hand...
- Inhale and slowly slide your right hand down to your ankles and hold the ankle if you can, or just place the hand on the side of the right leg.
- Keep your left arm close to the ear and look at the ceiling.
- Hold the position and slowly change to the other side.

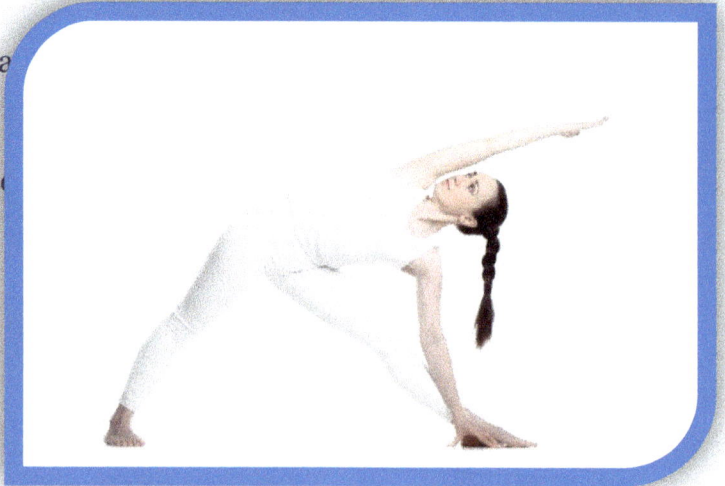

5. Angles pose 2:

- Stand tall and keep your legs one step apart from each other.
- Put your left hand on your waist and raise your right hand up.
- Inhale and slowly bend to the left side.
- Hold the pose for 10 seconds and cha...
- Repeat 3 times from both sides.

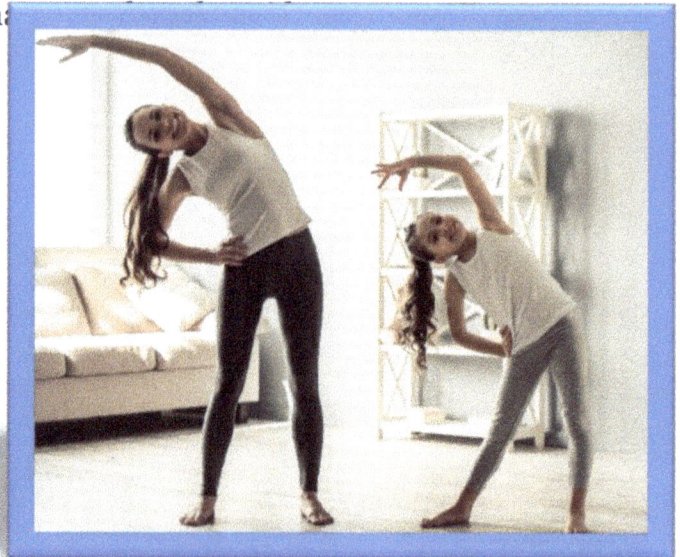

6. Chair pose:

- Stand tall and straight while keeping your legs apart and your back, neck straight.
- Raise your both arms in front
- Slowly bend your knees and sit like you are sitting on the chair.
- Hold the pose for 10 seconds.
- Repeat 3-5 times.

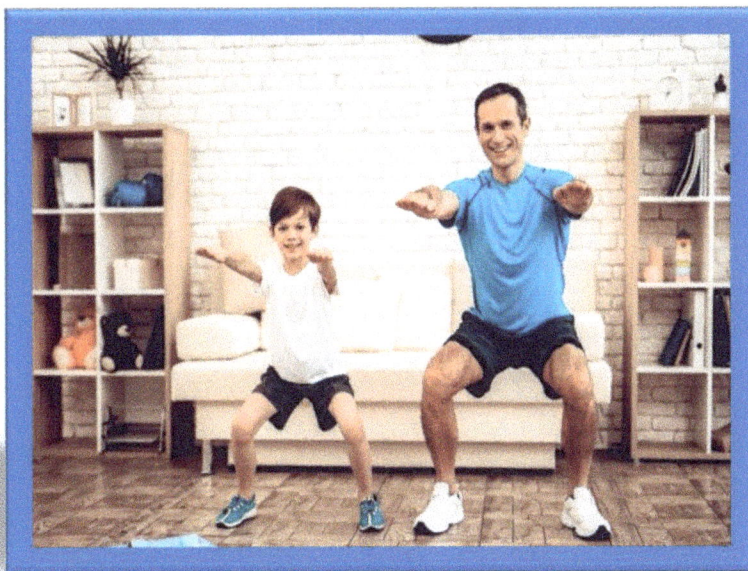

CHAPTER THREE

Yoga for Children - Improve Self Discipline

As the only time in your life when you were free from tension, stress and concern and the small world around you elicited your minimum needs, childhood remains fresh in your mind. It is a period when your body and mind are created and when your future behaviours and lifestyle are moulded. As a result, children are filled with energy. This is our role as a parent to channelise this energy in the right

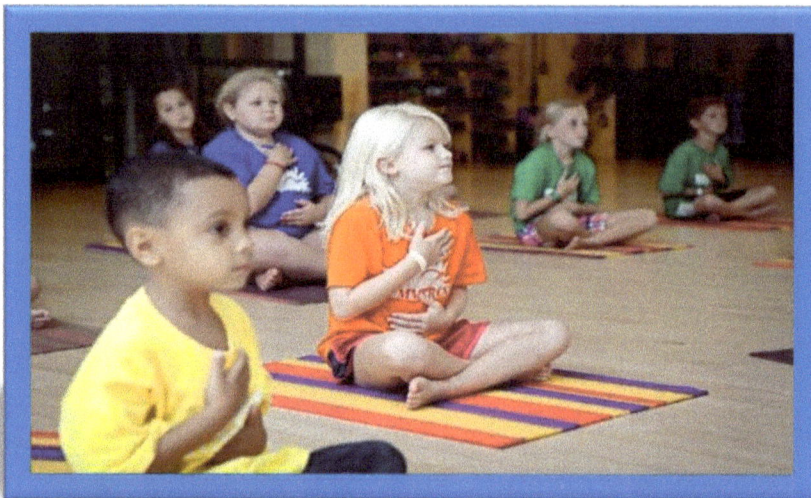

direction.

Our approach should guide our child's energy to the early practice of yoga to develop self-discipline and self-regulation.   Thus, the child strengthens his communication skills, respect for others, and his love and consideration for his fellow beings. In addition, yoga forms the coordination of strength, stability, flexibility, and balance of the child's body at this early age.

The practice of chanting Omkar, which allows even infants to listen to it, will increase children's attention and memory. Yoga Nidra(sleep) helps to increase the rapid release of sleeping growth hormone. The growth hormone plays a significant role in the fetus's development, and yoga Nidra plays a substantial role in the fusion and enhancement of the child's brain's separate developmental areas. The balancing postures often help to improve the child's attention and memory.

Excess levels of energy in Children

Most kids have excess energy at their age, which they convey with restlessness, and the child will end up with other problems unless you continue to guide it constructively. Proper breathing exercises will provide ample oxygen to the child's brain and body cells and bring about much-needed calm.

Short temper in kids

You can help solve children's problems with deep breathing. Pranayama and meditation interpret as a tool for adamant and short-tempered children. Yoga practice in a group or community will encourage a spirit of unity and teamwork; build a spirit of respect and a sense of love among the kids.

Every mother wants her kid to grow up tall and beautiful. Postures such as the triangle, fighter, mountain, tree pose, and Surya Namaskar (sun salutation) help increase the child's height in yoga and systematically stretch its spine and limbs to enhance its flexibility. Also, these postures assist in increasing the metabolism of calcium and its use in the body.

Respiratory concerns

Deep breathing exercises assessed in-depth help increase the supply of oxygen to the brain and cells. This helps prevent breathing issues such as cough and cold, asthma, bronchitis, etc.

Digestion Normally

Coupled with Surya Namaskar (a salute to the sun), preliminary yoga movements help increase metabolism and the mechanism of natural digestion, which increases the high immunity of the child's body to diseases.

Children appear to have an infinite energy supply. The practice of yoga helps children make more balanced use of their resources. A child who practices yoga gains the intensity and versatility of yoga practice. The clarity and calm of meditation help retain a connection with an inner sense of self, which is undoubtedly valuable when going through adolescence or teenage.

Historically, we have erred towards two extremes in raising our children: One, we have suppressed their energy in the quest for ways to control and socialise our children. Children have been exposed to long hours of school, where they are forced to sit on hard chairs and concentrate on what is being taught. Rigid demands and norms at home were also part of a normal upbringing which suppress the child's energy. The energy is moved outside the body, and the child is more vulnerable to the pickup of other energies in that state. Have you ever found that your child talks and behaves exactly like someone with whom they spend time? It means they have picked up their energy. The child's perception of him or herself becomes distorted. It also makes the body more susceptible to disease.

Kids did not have the discipline needed to learn self-discipline and good work habits. As a result, they have not learned to direct the tremendous energy they have provided as children. The energy conveys feelings that may not be in the child's best interest or the community. As a reaction from the first method, the sixties were a swing in this direction. The notion of 'I can do what I want' became famous in the sixties. Yet we forgot to ask, "what does the true me, the wisest I want to do?"

Asanas (postures) practice helps the child learn to direct their almost infinite energy supply, leading to improved physical, mental and emotional health. The classical asanas guide the child's energy in the body in a constructive, balanced way only by the shape of the asana. Each asana acts like a musical note's tonal sound or a perfect snowflake's crystalline form, helping to link the child with an element of their inner self. The practice of asanas helps to build in the body an atmosphere that is more welcoming to the child's true self.

By the age of seven, a child's nervous system is mature enough to begin yoga posture practice. Younger kids can start by incorporating the asanas with play to prepare their bodies and nervous systems. You will note how willingly the asana forms are folded into their bodies. If only we could preserve the marvellous versatility! The most successful form of yoga focuses on the careful alignment of the child's body until a child is mature enough to perform the asanas. An asana practice based on alignment helps improve strength and flexibility in a stable and balanced manner. But sitting in a meditation pose can be introduced at a very young age.

Meditation Practice teaches the child how to communicate with the mind and the body's natural energies. When a child learns to focus the mind's energy and body's life force, the child will start using this energy to communicate with the heart's inner teacher, resulting in a relaxed mind and a safe body.

The child learns how to contain their energy in the body if a child is brought up practising yoga and meditation. The child grows up with a stronger sense of self, starting to learn the art of establishing safe, balanced boundaries for the mind, body, and emotions. The unrelenting mainstream advertising would less attract children and less readily impacted by the popular culture tide. Based on what is best for them, they will be more likely to make choices. They grow up in the world with a greater sense of self, inner calmness, and a positive understanding of themselves. Hey, maybe their parents would even like to try it!

Yoga for improving self-discipline:

If you think your little one can start in this discipline and you want to guide or practice with them, we will present you with the best postures in a detailed list below.

1. Prayer posture

This posture is one of the first to execute when starting a yoga practice, as it helps to relax the body before beginning the session. To begin, the child should sit with crossed legs should be at a 90-degree angle with the little one should take several deep breaths inhaling and exhaling through the nose for three minutes.

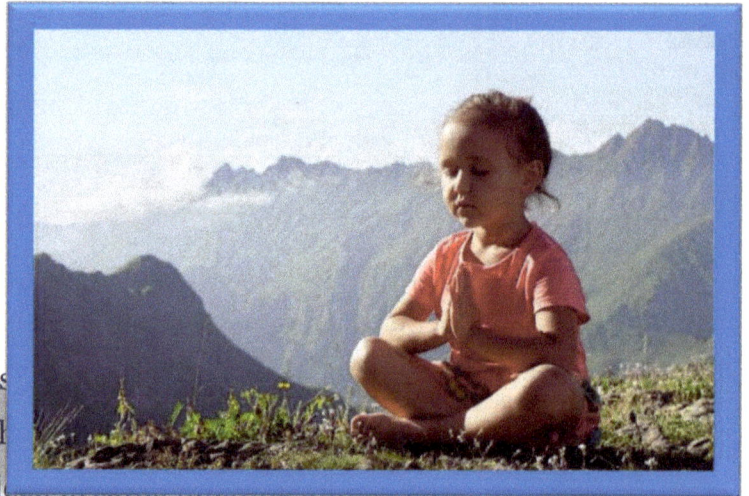

2. Butterfly pose:

1. The next position is the butterfly pose; this is one of the best yoga poses for children. With it, the child will begin to warm up and stretch his legs. The little one should sit with the legs bent, joining feet in the centre, and join palms in the namaskar pose.

24

2. Hold for a few seconds and move hands towards feet and then put your hands on your feet and move your legs up and down, emulating the movement of a butterfly's wings.

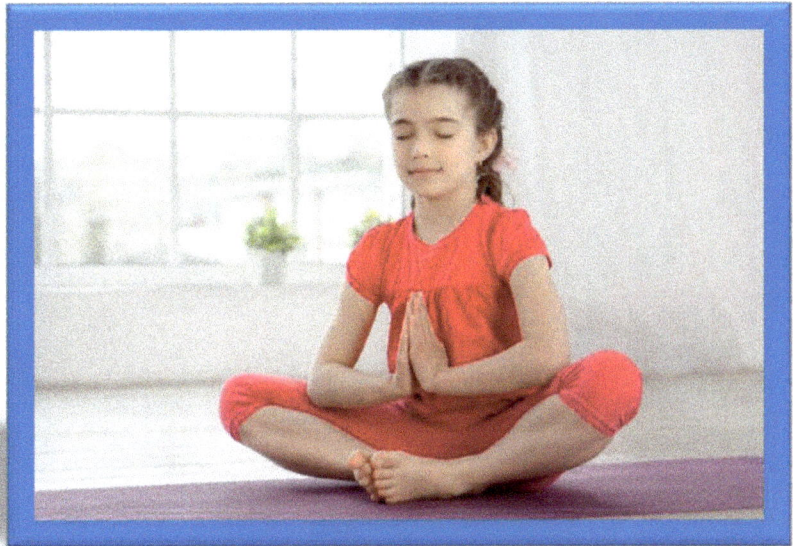

3. This pose is one of the most fun for little ones. They to do this movement unconsciously, even without being in a yoga class.

4. The recommended time before moving to the next position is 2 to 3 minutes.

3. Cobra pose

This pose is recommended to stretch the muscles of the abdominal and lumbar areas.

1. The child should lie on his yoga mat face down. Then place the palms on the ground at the side of the chest.

2. The next step will be to lift the body by stretching arms and curving back while looking up at the ceiling. This posture is contraindicated for children with spinal problems.

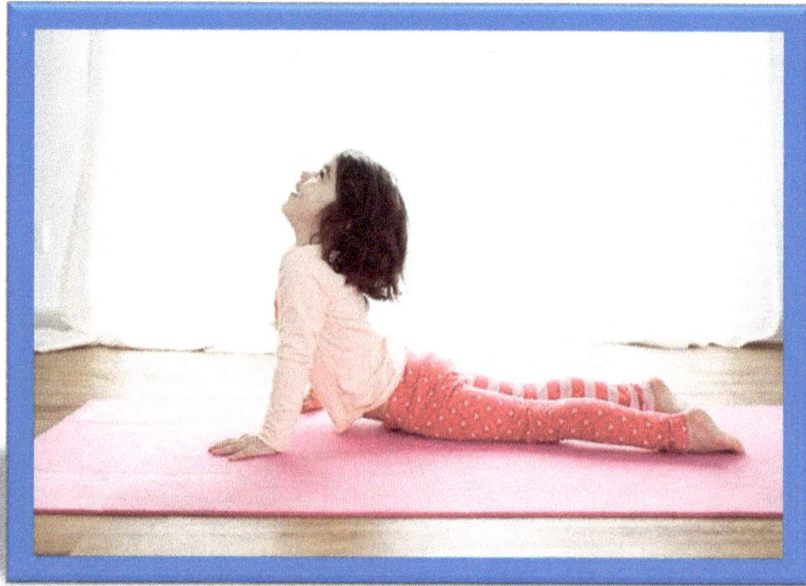

Once the child is master in all the above asanas, then Surya Namaskar can be introduced

7. **Salute to sun:** Surya Namaskar is a practice of yoga traditionally performed to warm up more challenging poses. The sun is the source of life and energy because this ancient yogi believed that worshipping the sun would lead to good health.

Surya Namaskar is an excellent warm-up for children because it stretches all the joints and major muscle groups. This smooth transition from poses helps one concentrate and focus and can have a marked effect on creativity. We will look at how to perform it.

Amazing benefits of Surya Namaskar:

The practice addresses parts of the body holistically, including most joints and major muscle groups. The poses and actions aid in toning the muscles of the body. The Surya Namaskar improves the child's body. The outer muscles and the inner muscles are trained. The practice can promote more than a hundred ailments. The main benefits of Surya Namaskar include:

- **Improved blood circulation:** There is a special focus on inhalation and exhalation, so the lungs are constantly ventilated. This means that, in a short time, the blood in the body is oxygenated and purified.
- **Increase fitness:** If the poses are carried out smoothly and fast, you will find the salute itself a great cardiovascular exercise. Excess weight around the stomach is easily trimmed off, and you can help your child be more active easily.
- **Benefits the skin and hair:** Activity improves blood circulation, so skin automatically becomes brighter and more radiant at a young age.
- **Anti-Anxiety:** Greeting helps children focus and improve their memory. It can have a great calming effect on the entire body. Any stress related to the exam or anything else can be eliminated by regularly practising the Surya Namaskar postures.
- **Optimised metabolism:** Another effect of the improved blood circulation is that; oxygen and nutrients reach all organs where needed, which means that the child's metabolism increases rapidly to optimal levels.

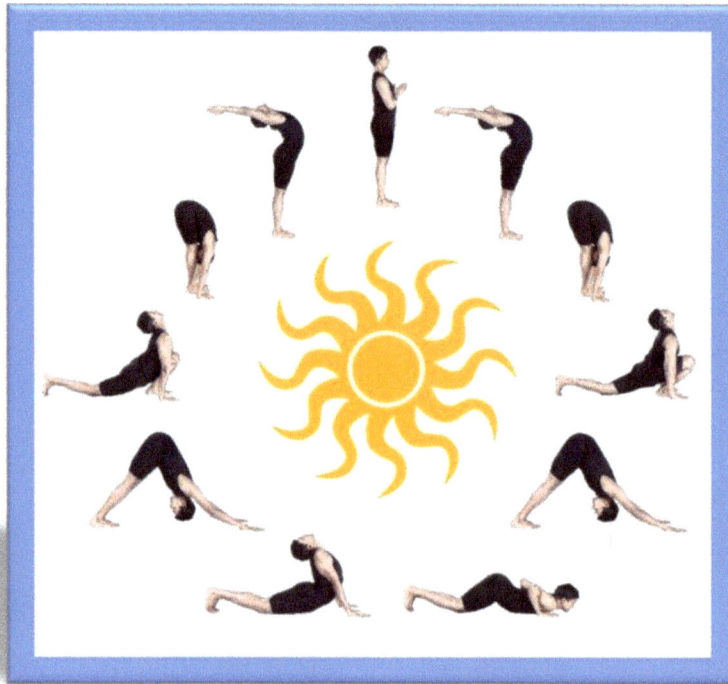

How to Make Surya Namaskar - A Step by Step Process

There are 12 asanas in the Surya Namaskar. Here is a detailed breakdown of the Surya Namaskar steps.

- **1. Pranamasana (Prayer posture)**
  Put your feet together and balance your weight on your feet equally. Expand your chest, and as you inhale, raise your arms on both sides, bring them together in front of the chest in the prayer position as you exhale.

- **2. Hasta Uttanasana (Raised arms pose)**
  Then inhale again and, with your biceps close to your ears, raise your arms up and back. Ensure that your entire body is stretched from your heels to your fingertips.

- **3. Hastapadasana (Standing forward bend)**
  Lean forward with your spine erect as you exhale and lower your hands to the ground next to your feet.

- **4. Ashwa Sanchalanasana (Lunge Pose)**
  Push your right leg back as far as possible while you inhale. Look up then and bring your right knee down to the ground.

- **5. Chaturanga Dandasana (Plank Pose)**

Similarly, with your body in a straight line and your arms perpendicular to the floor, take your left leg back as you inhale and go to the plank position.

- **6. Ashtanga Namaskar (Eight Limbed Pose)**
  Exhale and lie down with your knees together. Then bend your knees slightly and put them together. Next, raise your back slightly; eight points on the body - two hands, two feet, two knees, chest, and chin - should be the only points of contact between your body and the floor.

- **7. Bhujangasana (Cobra Pose)**
  Lift your chest with your elbows bent and your shoulder away from your ears. Stretch out as much as possible and make sure your chest pushes forward when you inhale. When you exhale, push your navel down gently.

- **8. Adho Mukha Svanasana (Downward-Facing Dog)**
  Lift your hips and tailbone with your palms still on the floor so that your body forms an inverted "V" shape. Make sure your heels touch the ground so your body remains straight.

- **9. Ashwa Sanchalanasana (Lunge Pose)**
  The inverted V returns to an equestrian stance with the right leg back and the chin facing up in one fluid motion. Stretch your body as much as possible.

- **10. Hastapadasana (Standing Forward Bend)**
  You should turn your legs' end and make them perpendicular with your hands by placing your hands on the floor above them.

- **11. Hasta Uttanasana (Raised Arms Pose)**
  Continuing the reverse trend, extend your spine as you exhale and raise your hands above your head. Stretch more instead of reaching back.

- **12. Pranamasana (Prayer Pose)**
  Exhale slowly, lower your arms and back to namaskar mudra and Relax and observe the various sensations that run through your body.

CHAPTER FOUR

Yoga for Children - Improve Self-Esteem

Over the last decade, we have witnessed a considerable increase in yoga from kindergartens, primary schools, and secondary schools, not only as a club activity after school but also as an essential part of its curriculum. More and more people see how yoga first-hand helps children. Mental health professionals, psychologists, neurologists, educators, and even the government begin to understand how yoga enhances children's mental wellbeing.

Yoga and mindfulness have many advantages, including learning, relaxation, stress release, and daily life support. For thousands of years, the art of yoga has been explored. There are vast benefits to the body and mind that have been observed and registered. However, the most significant effect of yoga is on a child's self-esteem. The sound of resonance and versatility inside the body and mind lifted. Their inner energy starts to flow like a calm river that crashes with the rough edges but still moves ahead in an aligned path.

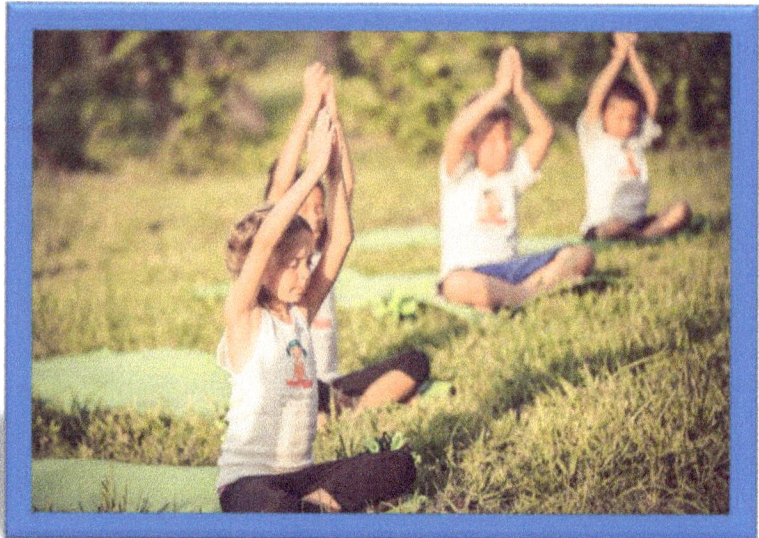

Mindfulness and psychological wellbeing

Mindfulness can help children learn to build up positive reactions to the unpredictable world around them. The technique's goal is to give the children the ability to control their thoughts by giving them the tools to focus on specific things. Mindfulness is undeniable when it comes to lowering stress that also boosts self-confidence.

Chakras will help kids learn at a deeper level about their social and emotional selves. Each of the seven chakras is aligned with the yoga poses below, combined with positive affirmations. In Yogic philosophy, the seven chakras represent seven endocrine glands important for our general health and develop the person's character. The aligning of these Chakras influence our body, mind, and soul.

In Sanskrit, each chakra, meaning "wheel", works as a spinning wheel of energy. Children and adolescents are not too young to understand chakras' fundamental principles, as the chakras grow throughout their lives. These poses of chakra yoga below will help them tune in to their wellbeing and fitness. Chakra yoga poses eventually help get the energy circulating across their bodies; building a balanced life may contribute to a deeper understanding of their holistic self.

CHAKRA POSES FOR KIDS: Try these poses with children and the pose-related affirmation and strengthen Chakras.

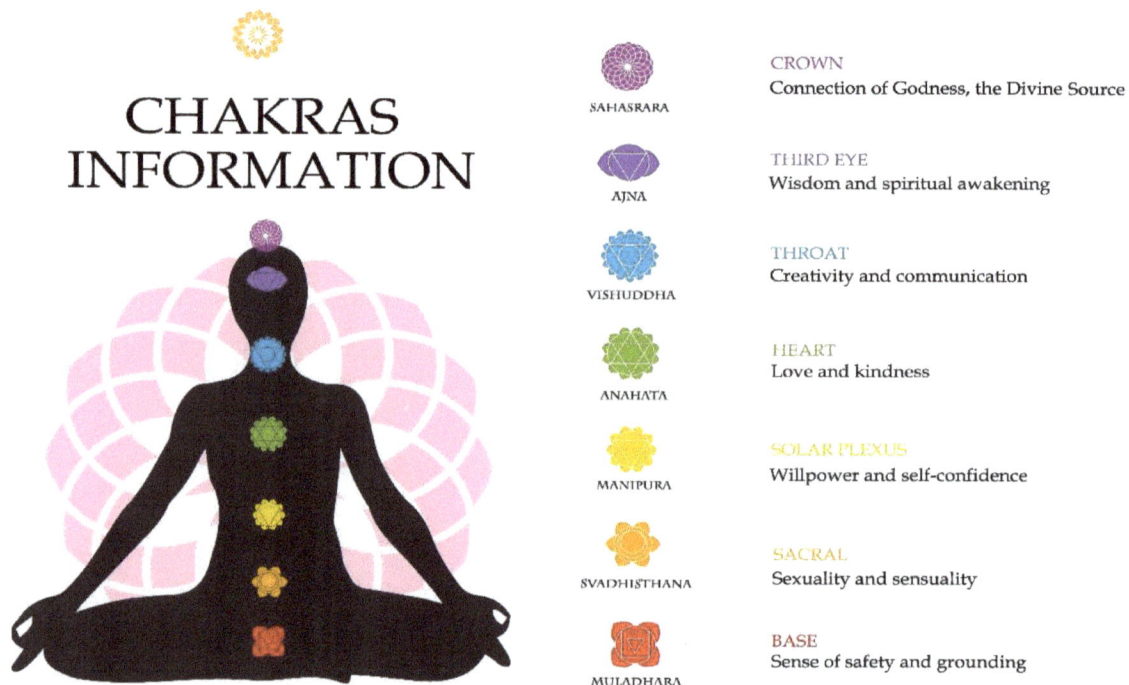

CHAKRAS INFORMATION

CROWN
Connection of Godness, the Divine Source

SAHASRARA

THIRD EYE
Wisdom and spiritual awakening

AJNA

THROAT
Creativity and communication

VISHUDDHA

HEART
Love and kindness

ANAHATA

SOLAR PLEXUS
Willpower and self-confidence

MANIPURA

SACRAL
Sexuality and sensuality

SVADHISTHANA

BASE
Sense of safety and grounding

MULADHARA

FIRST CHAKRA – Muladhara Chakra - I am healthy

Tadasana: PalmTree Pose: Stretching the body activates chakras, especially the Muladhara chakra, based around the tail bone.

This asana will teach how to maintain proper body posture.

- Stand with your feet parallel, slightly apart. Feel the soles of your feet as the union of your being with the earth. Feel your weight on them, make sure that your weight is balanced equally on both feet. Unlock your knees.

- Interlock your fingers, Inhale, raise your arms above your head with palms facing towards the ceiling.

- Stretch your body as much as you can on your tiptoes whilst keeping your back straight.

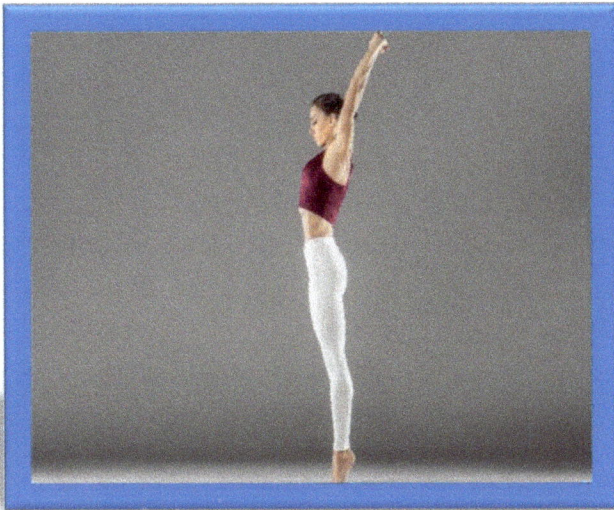

- The abdominal area should maintain a slight tension.

- Exhale and slowly back to your normal position by leaving the arms loose at the sides of the body.

- Repeat 3-5 times.

SECOND CHAKRA – Swadhisthan Chakra - I Love my life

Half Moon Pose:

- Drive your left foot out back from a standing position while opening your hip to the side. Tilt forward and put your right hand flat in front of your rig simultaneously raising your left f up to the ceiling. Align and ope

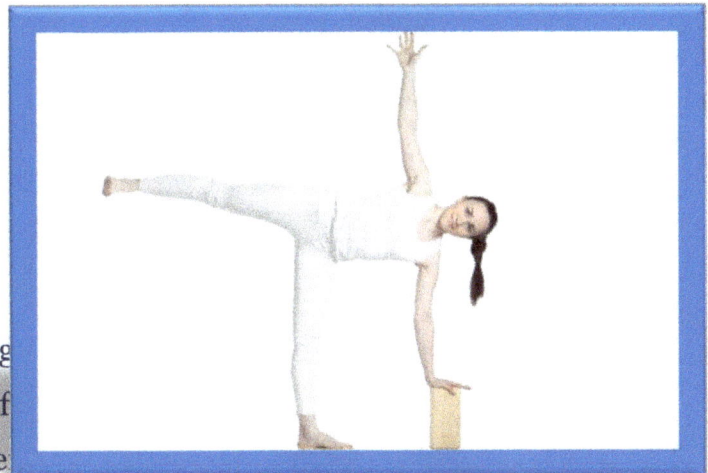

other. Try looking out to the left, if possible. Repeat the measures by flipping sides.

THIRD CHAKRA – Manipura Chakra - I Believe in Myself

Wall Pose (Viparita Karani):

Initially, this asana can be started with the support of the wall.

•Lie down on the floor and lift legs with the wall's support until hips touch the wall.

•Try to keep legs straight at 90°. Hold the position for 5 minutes.

•When they become confident in holding their legs and body, They can do with the support of their hands instead of the

•Slowly try to bring legs towards the head and try to touch the floor

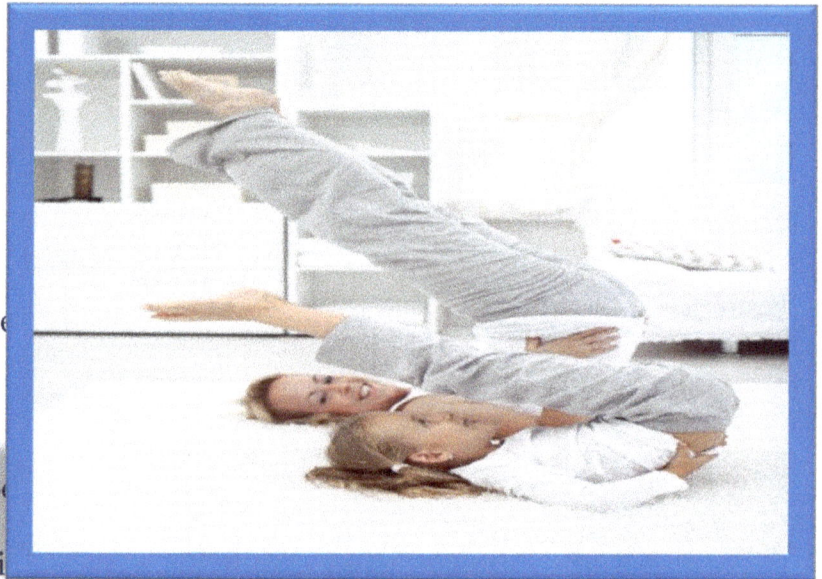

This pose improves blood circulation, insomnia, reduces the tension of lower back and tired feet, and relaxes pelvic floor muscles.

FOURTH CHAKRA – Anahata Chakra – I am creative.

Bridge Pose:

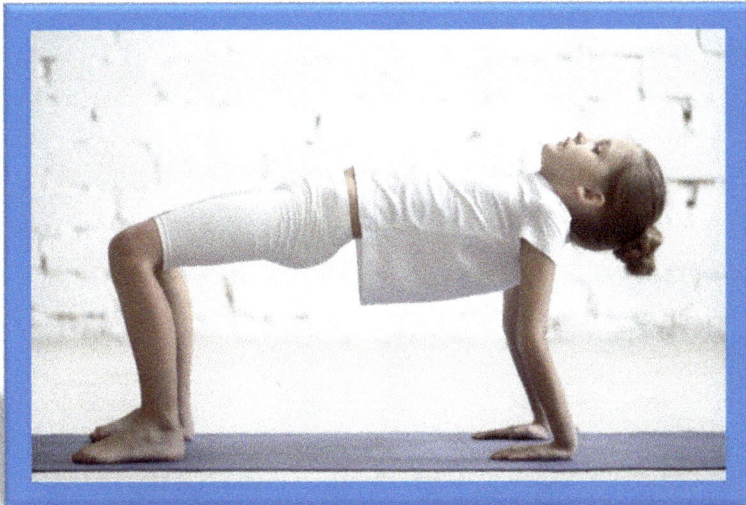

- With your k n e e s bent and your feet flat on the mat, lie on your back.
- Rest your arms flat on the ground alongside your body, with your palms flat.
- Keep your spine straight, tuck your head into your stomach.

- Raise your buttocks as you inhale, keeping balance your body on your arms and legs, hold the posture for 20 seconds, exhale slowly bring your body down on the mat.
- Repeat 3-5 times.

FIFTH CHAKRA – Vishudha Chakra - I stay positive and alert. **Down dog Pose:**

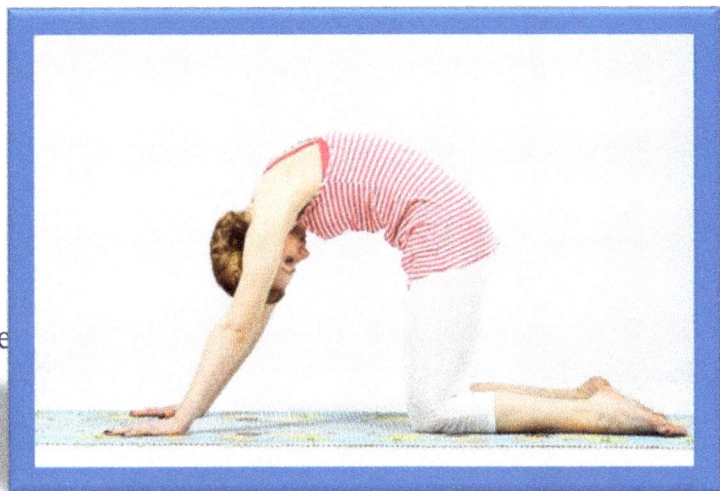

- Place your hands in front of you, from all fours, while dropping your chest to the

- Hold your arms upright and lift your elbows off the ground.
- Rest your forehead between your extended arms, tuck your tummy in and naturally allowing your spine to curve.

SIXTH CHAKRA – Ajna Chakra - I am OPEN-MINDED.

Camel pose: Sit in vajra asana, hold your ankles with yourhands, and slowly stretch your body. Look at the ceiling; maintain the posture if you can.

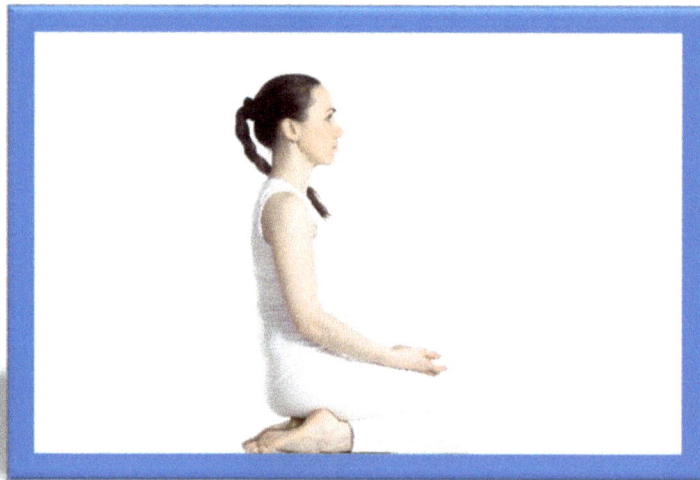

Vajra Asana

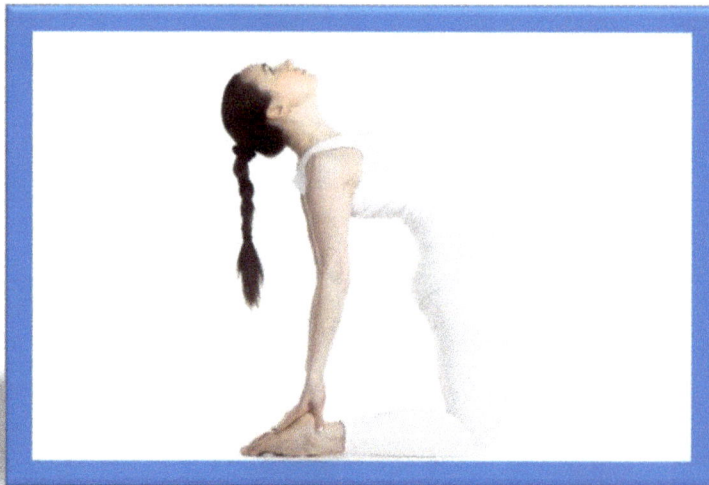

Camel Pose

SEVENTH CHAKRA – Sahastarar Chakra - I am peaceful.

Corpse (Resting)Pose:

- Lie with your arms and legs spread out on your side in a comfortable position.
- Close your eyes and focus on the centre of your forehead between two eyebrows. Keep doing a deep breath in and out for 10 minutes.

If a child is having problems focusing on the centre of the forehead, use sandalwood powder (mix with water and make a paste), put it at the centre of the forehead.

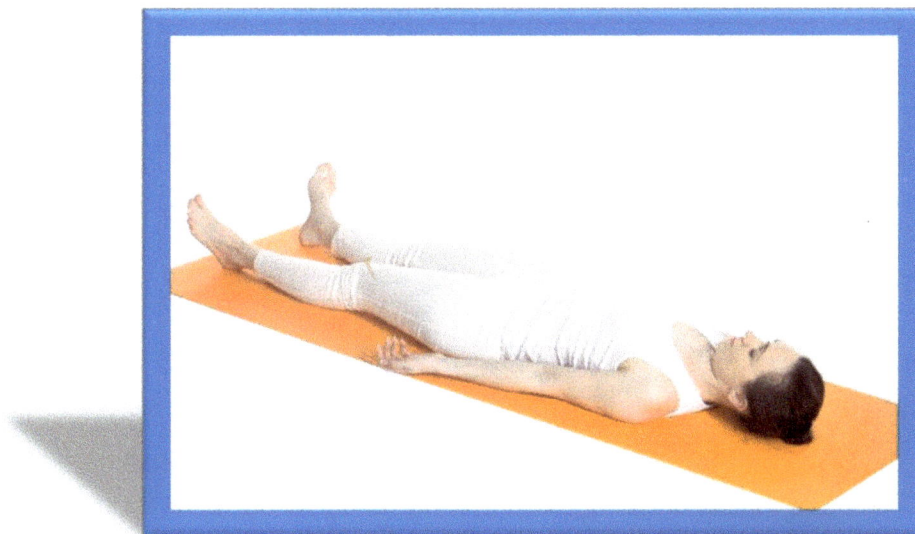

CHAPTER FIVE

Yoga for Children - Improve Self-Concentration

The mind of a child is more versatile than an adult. Thus, to adapt to new developments, it is simple to train.

However, what you train and how you train your child makes the difference between making oneself an aware individual and not.

You need your child to be able to restrict both the mind and the body to enhance focus. So, you need to begin by teaching the basic poses of yoga.

Children get the opportunity to focus better by practising yoga as their nervous and cardiovascular systems are controlled.

Yoga also helps balance hormones and provides the child with a relaxed body to focus and concentrate.

Yoga encourages your child to eternally living a balanced life and increases the ability to respond.

How to teach children yoga

It is not easy to teach children yoga. Still, suppose you are a regular and disciplined person. In that case, you can easily make yoga and mindfulness a part of your children's lifestyle. Then, you need to start practising yoga yourself and do it with consistency.

Start by waking up at a set time and getting the kids up. This time needs to be at least half an hour before the specified time to practice yoga.

On the other hand, if you are a person who can spend time with your children in the evening, you might turn the yoga session into an evening and make it a routine.

Yoga should be done systematically to bring about mind conditioning, which will improve children's memory and imagination.

Out of all the yoga postures that a child can perform, many of them are especially great for enhancing their energy and concentration.

Kids are fast learners, and you can easily see how quickly they pick up yoga and mindfulness as part of their lives.

As a rule, beginning with simple, easy to follow, and successful postures, you can slowly find that both you and your child can shift to complex poses.

The first thing that comes up when asking how to boost children's attention is to sit quietly in a position with specific yoga mudras or movements that are the steppingstone to mindfulness.

For this, follow the steps below.

- Position yourself with crossed legs (Padmasana) and join the palms together.
- Keep the back straight as you take deep breaths.
- Close your eyes and relax.
- Now bring your hands together behind your back. Then, hold opposite wrists.
- As slowly as you can, bend forward and touch the ground with the top of your head.
- Breathe out while bending.
- Sit for a short period in that specific position and then slowly return to the starting position.
- It should be repeated five times.

Benefits

- Fills the body with energy and vitality
- Boosts memory power

This is the best way to start a day. Done early in the morning.

Salamba sarvangasana for kids

The candle position (salamba Sarvangasana) is one of the healthiest yoga exercises that offer many therapeutic benefits. It is not the simplest one, and many experienced yogis consider it the crowning achievement o f yoga practice. Nevertheless, i t is worth doing the candle position bec many ailments, dysfunctions

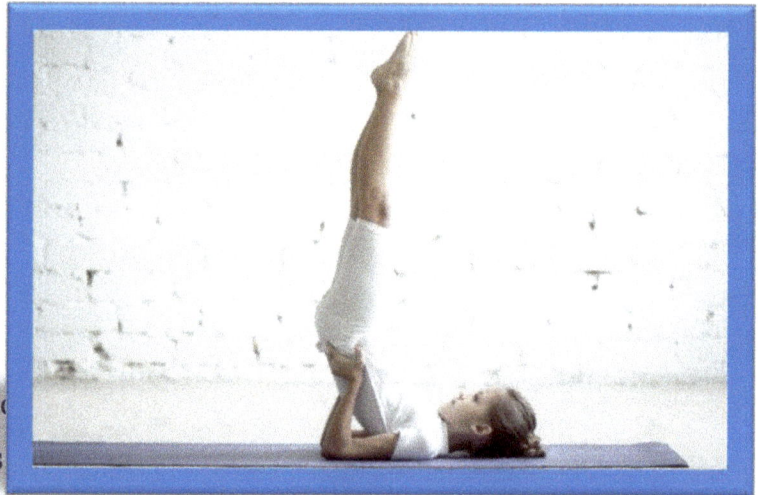

The candle (salamba Sarvangasana) is called the lunar position. This means that it is a passive position. To perform it, one must adopt an appropriate, inverted position of the body and stay in it as long as possible, relaxing the muscles as possible and leading to a feeling of rest. It will not be easy at first, but practice makes perfect!

The candle position is excellent for your mental and physical health, which means that making a candle has many benefits for your body and soul.

You can help your child by holding their legs up.

How to make a candle - step by step instruction

- Fold the blanket or mat until it is rectangular and protects the shoulders well against the hard ground.
- Lie down so your head is on the floor and your shoulders and back are on the blanket.
- Place your hands at your hips and bend your legs.
- Now, pushing yourself off the floor with your hands, lift your torso, keeping your legs bent.
- Correct your hand position to support your back well. Try to get the torso position as straight as possible and bring your chin closer to your chest so that it rests on the collarbone and is as close as possible to the sternum.
- Then slowly stretch your legs up. Do not tense your face or throat muscles. Keep your position straight at all costs. Do not let your legs drop down towards your chest and your lumbar spine sagging. Keep your elbows close and your legs and arms symmetrically. You can help your child initially for holding the position.
- Hold this position for five minutes. Then increase its duration to seven minutes or even fifteen minutes.
- When practising a candle, remember that this is a position in which your body should rest. If you have joint pain or too much pressure in your eyeball or throat, stop. Practice and regularity will ensure that, if you do not have any severe health constrictions for candle exercise, over time, you will be able to endure this influential yoga position for longer and longer.
- **Benefits of a candle:** The candle is one of the most influential yoga poses. It gives a lot of benefits, not only physical but also pro-health. This is because the candle ranks among the inverted lunar positions. It is

performed passively, which gives our body energy that calms, relaxes, and tones.

Bhujapidasana :

- Sit in a squatting position. Place your feet at a distance slightly less than shoulder-width and keep your knees wide open.

- Fold your legs forward until your torso is between your inner thighs. Put your hands inside your feet and make sure elbows touching the inside of your knees. Try to put your weight forward.

- Place your shoulders underneath the thighs placing your hands flat on the ground on your feet' outsides. The heels of hands should align with the heels of the feet. This will make your upper back curve.

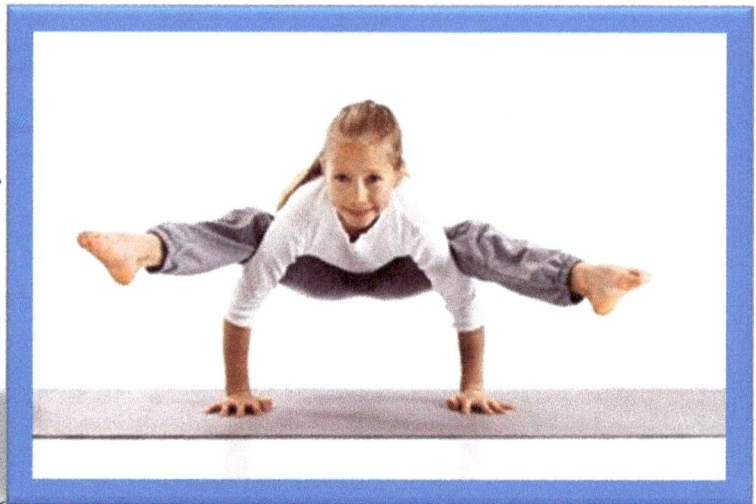

- Press your palms firmly on the ground, slowly lift your feet up off the floor

- Hold the pose for 20 seconds or as long as comfortable. Slowly return to your starting position by bending your elbows and releasing your feet back to the floor.

Pranayama Yoga:

Pranayam Yoga is the best when it comes to improving concentration and attention span. Prana means – breath, life force, energy, and Yama mean discipline. The actual meaning is the discipline of life force that is breathing.

Controlling the breath is the ultimate therapy for physical and mental wellbeing. If we discipline our children to sit daily in meditation and focus on breathing, that will help them focus and improve concentration.

Here, some pranayama yoga can be introduced to boost memory and create space for new learning and improve overall mental power.

1.Deep breathing exercise I:

- Sit in a meditation pose and deep breath through your nose with the expansion of your chest.
- Slowly breath out through your nose with your mouth closed.
- Only use the nose for this breathing exercise.
- Repeat 3-5 times (or until you feel settled or calm).

2. Deep breathing exercise II:

- Sit in a meditation pose and deep breath through your nose.
- Curl your lips like a whistle.
- Breathe out slowly through your mouth.
- Repeat 3-5 times.

3.Deep Breathing exercise III:

- Sit in a meditation pose and deep breath through your nose.
- Bring your hand in front of your chest and join your fingertips and thumbs of both hands.
- Control your breath while closing your fingers and thumbs in and opening fingers and thumbs while breathing out.
- Close your eyes and repeat five times.

4.Anulom Vilom:

This exercise has magical power and unlimited benefits. This exercise only connects directly to the brain; it relaxes the brain in a few minutes. Anulom-Vilom is a combination of Lunar and solar breathing. That means it regulates the body temperature and keeps us healthy in all seasons. This exercise is done like this:

- Close your right nostril, inhale through the left nostril. Hold the air. Close your left and exhale to the right.
- Now close the left nostril, inhale from the right. Hold the air. Close your right nostril and exhale to the left.
- Keep your eyes closed and focus on your brain; maintain your rhythm for 10-15 minutes.
- While focusing on your brain, imagine that the positive energy is going into your brain and deleting all negative, sad, corrupt, unwanted and junk files of your brain.
- The most significant benefit of this exercise is that you cannot think anything else when maintaining the rhythm(cycle).

This Pranayama Yoga increases positivity and helps to get rid of negative thoughts.

It refreshes, reboots and restarts the brain for new learning.

It promotes overall wellbeing and improves the ability to focus and concentrate.

5.Bhramari Pranayam:

This is Bramari, the "buzzing bee" pranayama, so named because the sound you make when you breathe resembles a black bee buzzing sound.

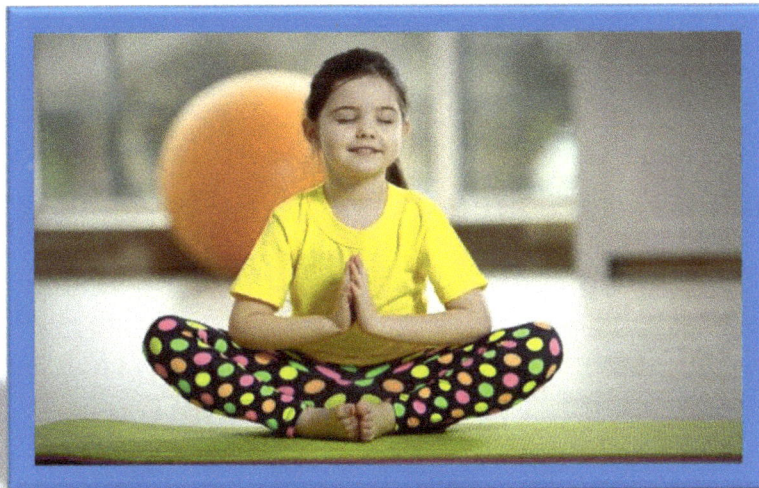

Brahmari pranayama:

- Sit in any comfortable meditative posture, relax your body.

- While sitting in meditation pose, keep your back and neck straight, join both hands at the centre in namaskar mudra, deep breath in and breath out with buzzing sound.

- Second technique - Place your thumbs in your ears (pressing the ear tubercle's middle outer part against the ear opening to completely block the ears), three fingers on the eyes and one finger on the forehead.

- Breath-in and then breath-out with buzzing Om sound. Remember to keep your mouth closed. Try to repeat five times. In Bhramari, the vibration sound produced is very soothing, so this practice eases mental tension and anxiety and helps reduce irritability.

Attention and Attention Spans in Young Children

One of the most important keys to success in school is having a well-developed focus period. For this, it is important to understand what attention is. In this way, you will help your children and better understand their concentration and attention span necessary for their educational and personal development.

Children can sometimes have difficulty concentrating in class, which can cause them to miss out on learning opportunities and not keep up with their classmates.

It can be challenging to solve a concentration problem when a child is already 8 or 9 years old. The best time to work on this skill is during the first years of life, when you, as a parent, can actively develop concentration and attention span.

What is the attention span?

The attention span or concentration is the child's ability to pay full attention to a specific task. It requires blocking out all other stimuli, such as sound (the class next door makes a noise), pictures (seeing what happens on the other side of the window), or unnecessary information (irrelevant writing on the board).

During the school day, children need to repeatedly focus on different tasks in an environment that can be very stimulating.

So, monitor your child's attention span during their preschool years and make sure it increases slowly over time. The school will become challenging and exhausting for a child who has difficulty concentrating.

It is easier to develop in the preschool years than later in life, as with all other skills. In this sense, it is essential to help children, through play and fun, to practice their attention span.

What is the average attention span of a pre-schooler?

The average attention span and concentration for a pre-schooler is typically less than 15 minutes. That is, 15 minutes purely focused on a task. For younger pre- schoolers, it is 5 minutes. As they grow older, they can focus longer. Generally, half an hour is appropriate in the first courses.

If you are concerned about your child's ability to concentrate, you first must ask yourself if you expect him to concentrate for a manageable period. It is much more effective to work on short tasks and provide frequent breaks than to try to sit for an hour with a 4-year-old.

A great way to refocus your child during an activity is to try quick mental breaks, such as mindfulness or yoga activities, which will allow them to relax their body and mind simultaneously.

Children's days at school are structured. They are taught in short periods with regular changes in the types of activities.

Quick exercises to improve attention spans in children

Next, we will explain some exercises that will be useful for you to do with your children and improve their attention spans. They are quick to do and easy to remember. Children will have a great time, and you just must give them little instructions. If you do it with them, so much, the better!

- Sitting exercises
- Sit with your legs stretched out in front of your children.
- Shake your legs.

- Roll your feet inward and outward.
- Stretch your toes forward.
- Stretch your toes back.
- Press knees down on the mat, hold for a few seconds and release.
- Bend over and hold your toes.

Standing exercises to improve attention spans

- Move your arms up and down to the sides, like a flying bird.
- Shrugs your shoulders. Shrug one shoulder at a time, forward andt h e n back. Then shrug both shoulders together, front and then back.
- Swing your arms back and forth.
- Swing your arms out to the sides like a windmill. Make small rotations first, then wider rotations. Start with one arm at a time and then both arms at the same time.

Walking exercises

- Walk backwards with small steps and then significant steps.
- Walk sideways, first to the right, then to the left.
- Imagine that you are walking on a rope. Go straight.

Balance exercises

- Stand on one leg. Count to 5, then switch and stand on the other leg.
- Stand on the tips of your toes. When you are in balance, close your eyes and stand on tiptoe.
- Again, stand on your toes and walk across the room.
- Jump with your feet together, then one foot at a time.

Lying down exercises to improve attention spans

- Pretend to be a ball. Hold your knees tightly. Pretend to be a ball and rock back, forward, and around.

- Sliding seal. Lie face down. Stretch your arms towards your back and fold your legs. Hold your ankles with your hands and slide side to side.

- Next, keep your legs straight, stretch your arms in front of the head, interlock your fingers, stretch your hands, and lift your head, chest, and legs up.

- Flying plane. Lie face down. Raise your arms and keep them in the air like an aeroplane. Then move your arms up and down.

Simple Exercises to Help Your Child Improve Attention

Improving attention is one of the most frequent challenges that parents face every day with their children. Suppose we start to put into practice the recommended exercises to help improve in this aspect. In that case, the results can favour this process and the relationship between parents and children.

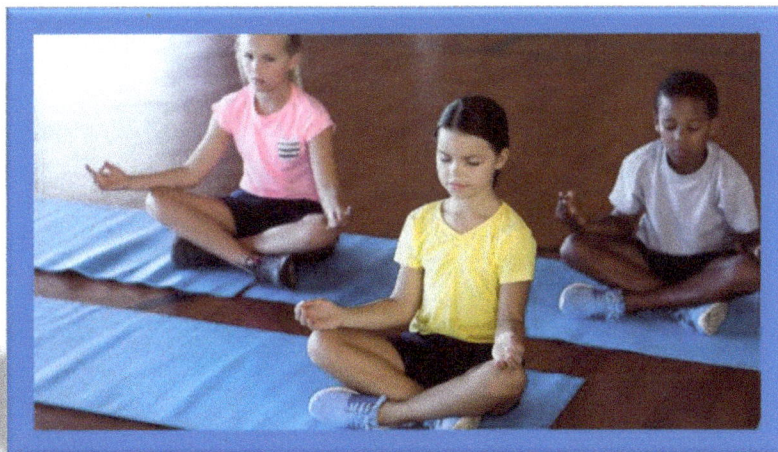

Sometimes, the lack of attention is a more serious problem than we can think. Each mother's desire is for her children to overcome this situation so that it is not linked to their adulthood attention deficit related to any element that slows down the process.

How to recognise the attention deficit?

This is a behavioural disorder that is directly affiliated with hyperactivity. In this way, it is possible to notice that our children are a little "hyperactive" or unruly.

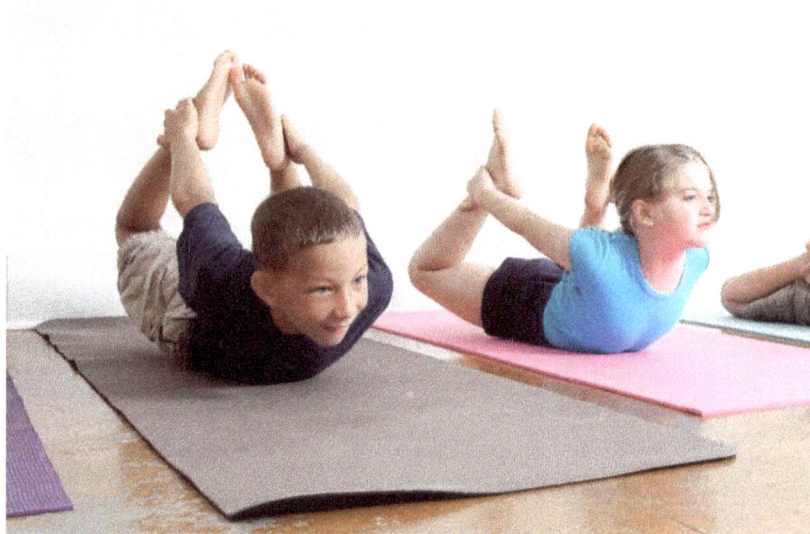

Children who are in this situation usually show the following signs:

- They do not seem to listen when addressed directly to them
- Does not keep a joke for long
- They tend to make mistakes in school because they miss some details
- Have organisational difficulties
- They are uncomfortable with activities that imply the intense mental ability
- Do not finish tasks or get confused with instructions.
- Are likely to lose valuables

If we quickly execute actions designed to solve any problem for our children, we are guaranteed to achieve good results.

Steps to Improve Your Children's Attention

- It begins by helping you set clear goals and objectives: the best thing in these cases is to set short-term objectives. This makes it mandatory to plan appropriately. Also, the results can be achieved quickly.

- Try to create a suitable environment: sometimes parents make distractions in children, so we must avoid overloading environments with possible distractors.

- Identify the cause of inattention: we may believe that a specific element of our environment should not be a source of distraction for children, but the smallest object will likely lead to disinterest in their work. Try to identify the item and eliminate it immediately.

- Keep what you need close at hand: avoid neglecting the child in his tasks because you have not gathered all the resources. This causes a setback in the activity because the child can lose his attention very quickly.

- Reinforce their confidence: avoid using words that can make them stop their interest. Remember always make positive comments about their performance and, at the same time, allow them to reinforce themselves.

- Locate the correct space: ensure that the area has the optimal conditions and bring it to this place all the time. Remember that if you change space frequently, the child will start again from zero in his observation.

- Take control with love: if your child has shown the signs of inattention, it is time for you to take control of their activities, as long as you respect their space. Never forget that your child will commit to better behaviour as long as you are firm and loving.

CHAPTER SIX
Yoga for Children - Improve Self-Motivation

Yoga is known as an act of talking with the inner self. A "Be Well" conversation during the Yoga session each morning will prepare children for new learning on a new day.

It is easy to motivate children to do the desired task; you just need to know their interests and how they like to be treated. Children often follow their parent's advice and listen to their parents. Still, initially, you must lure them with their favourite thing.

Once the habit of doing yoga every day, a ritual and a positive energy build-up inspire them to keep moving forward, following the rituals.

You have noticed that if there was a ritual at your home that you were following from your childhood and you keep doing that ritual and feel anxious if you cannot do it.

The habits are formed in childhood, and we carry them our whole life until some sweeping change happens to our lives.

Here are some tips to motivate your children and make a habit of yoga every day.

- Yoga time should be short, fun, and enjoyable.
- Do yoga with your children; incorporate it as a family ritual.
- Give them time to settle first; as a parent, you start doing it and ask them to sit with you.
- Start some funny and exciting yoga pose challenges between siblings and yourselves.

- Empower them with benefits and start noticing the changes in height, weight, and behaviours.

- A reinforcement chart can be used or paste smiley face stickers on the calendar for every new achievement.

- Motivate them for doing 5 sets of yoga asanas to get their favourite game, toy, or dinner.

- If the game is costly and dinner is not a healthy option, use the sticker technique. Children have to achieve a certain number of stickers, e.g., 30- 50, so they stick to it, and you will get time to move on to other reinforcement.

- A healthy competition between the siblings is ideal for getting up early, arranging the yoga room, lighting the candle in the yoga room, etc.

- According to *Psycho-Cybernetics,* a book published by plastic surgeon Maxwell Maltz in 1960, it takes 21 days to make a habit or second human nature. But it depends on person to person.
  Some Individuals take more time, and some take less than 21 days, but the main thing is that you must stick with it to convert it into your and your children second nature.

- Celebrating children's achievements plays a vital role in motivation. Try to celebrate their 10 days or 21 days achievements according to their interest.

- Never arrange a yoga session when a child is tired or just turned off the video game.

    Our body and mind are interconnected. Our body passes the signals to the brain through our senses. Our brains read these senses and respond accordingly. Suppose if our senses are giving signals as a threat to life and show any danger and stress. In that case, the brain sends stress signals and produces hormones to prepare the body for fight and flight situations. For example, while playing violent video games, children are constantly sending the fight and flight signal to the brain; if they lose the game, their heartbeat increases, faces and body are tightened. Because the brain starts producing hormones needed to get away from that situation, it makes them restless and aggressive. (The article published in science direct). The day-to-day issue can incorporate their roles too. Stay positive in diverse life situations can be challenging for anyone and especially for children.

- On the other hand, Positive energy is subtle energy, so the brain cannot read it as a threat and react calmly. Negative energy shakes the brain, and the body responds accordingly. It is hard to motivate children to sit for yoga or meditation at that time. Let their mind settle in, body calm down.

- Feel good factor is essential if you try to introduce new habits or motivate your child to develop the second nature.

Yoga for Children by Age

Many situations can cause anxiety and stress in children. Given this, we must know what techniques to use so that the little ones relax.

Benefits of Yoga for children by age

Yoga and relaxation are not only good for adults, but it is also good for children. So let us see some benefits of using these techniques:

- Decrease the level of anxiety.
- Stop stuttering.
- Prevents asthmatic attacks.
- Improves the quality and problems of sleep.
- Increases the quality of the child's learning.
- Decreases the frequency of nervous tics.
- Improves concentration and memory.
- Improvements, in general, in the wellbeing of the little ones.
- Reduces muscle tension.
- It helps control emotions, especially in those cases in which children have outbursts of anger and aggressiveness.

For babies from 1 to 3 years

At these ages, ' children can participate less, so we will use yoga poses to help them enjoy sitting with you.

Shantala massage technique consists of stimulating, relaxing, and helping children to relax through touch. It is essential to do these massages when the baby is calmer, not in the middle of a tantrum. We can help them with calm and soft music, dim lighting, and adequate room temperature.

This is a perfect age to start developing habits and let children know that this is a part of life. You can begin yoga by massaging their feet, legs, stomach, back, chest, arms, and hands and doing some exciting poses that a child can perform.

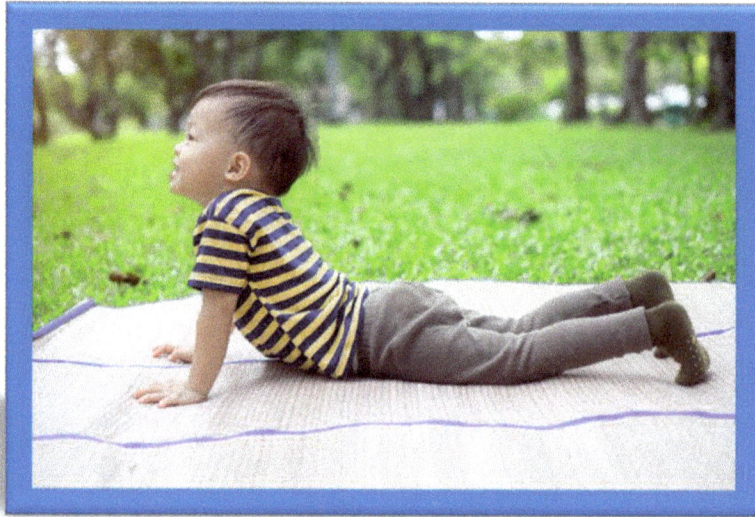

For children from 3 to 7 years

In this stage, the participation of children is more active than in the previous one.

Turtle pose:

Sit with open legs, stretch both legs in a comfortable position, bend forward, e x t e n d your arms, place your head on the floor, or place your han

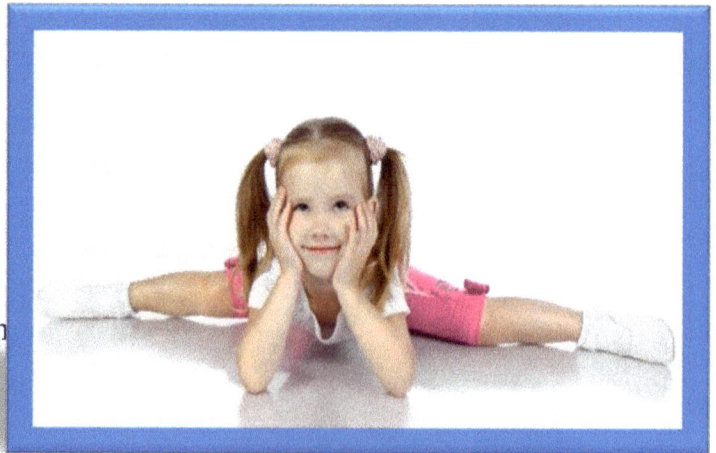

Child Sitting Triangle Pose:

Sit with a straight back and stretch your right leg and fold your left leg so that the left foot is touching the right thigh. Now extend your right arm and touch the toes of your right leg. Hold the pose for 2 minutes and change, do the same with another leg.

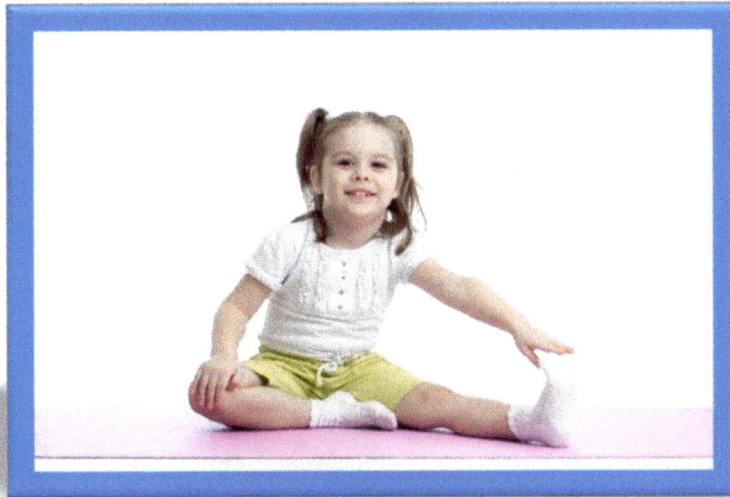

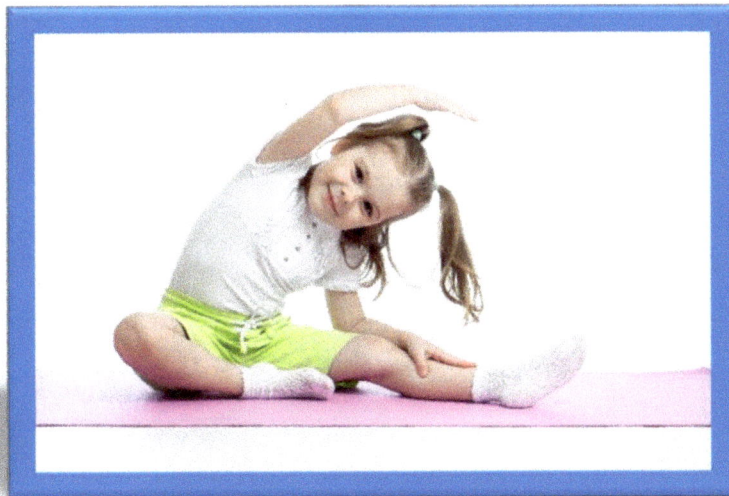

For children from 7 to 9 years

These children already have better control over themselves. Therefore, we can use some m o r e complicated poses like – Surya Namaskar, pigeon pose, camel pose, and other balancing poses.

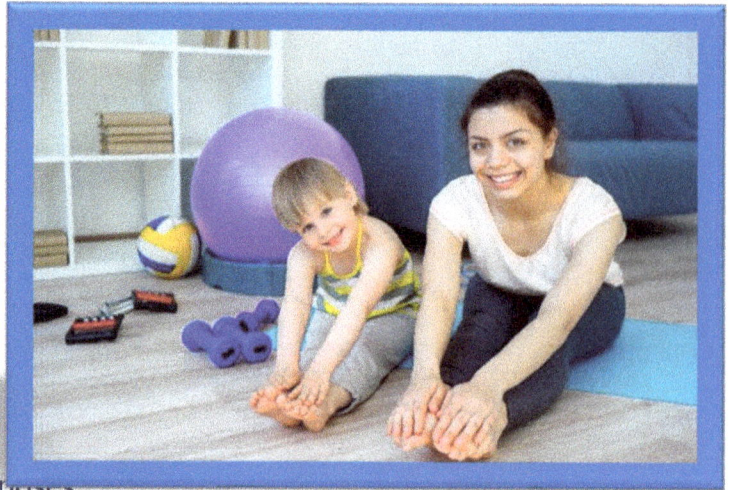

For children from 9 to 12 years old: At these ages, we can use any technique that helps the child relax and can do it in any situation in which he feels nervous, such as an exam. One of the methods that we can use is Pranayama Yoga. Also, if children practise it frequently, it will be effortless to do it when needed.

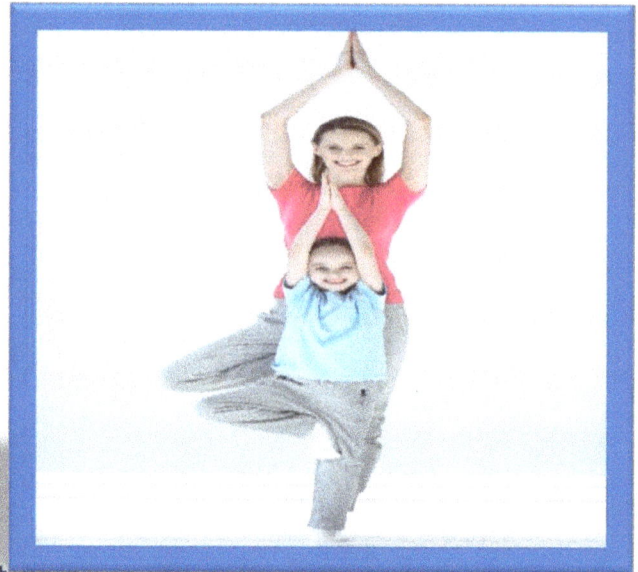

This consists of tensing the different parts of the body for 10 seconds and then gently relaxing them. Breathing will be done by inhaling deeply for a few seconds and exhaling slowly. Use the code 6-2-7, inhale to six, hold your breath for two and exhale to 7.

Yoga with Teens:

Let us break down why yoga is beneficial for Teens as we explore their colourful and turbulent world.

Physical Fitness

The adolescent years can roughly be divided into th

- 1: Early adolescence- 11-13 years
- 2: Middle adolescence- 14-16 years
- 3: Late adolescence- 17-21 years

Teens put on an impressive growth spurt between the ages of 11 and 21 to help them achieve their final adult height, boys and girls grow up very quickly, and it is clumsy, their body grows so fast that their brains can rapid growth surge is caused by higher testosterone sex hormone levels, which also causes the sexual organs to develop, a sign that your teen is undergoing puberty.

The shapeshift for girls means that oestrogen causes the laying down of fat, cycles begin, and the pelvis widens in preparation for childbirth to become smooth. Bones become denser and thicker for boys as the muscle fibres lengthen and expand, the chest and shoulders extend. As you can see, a lot is going on, and during this time, teenagers can experience physical distress from growing pain (as bones grow), acne, more sweating, period pain (for girls), a crack in the vocal cords (for boys),

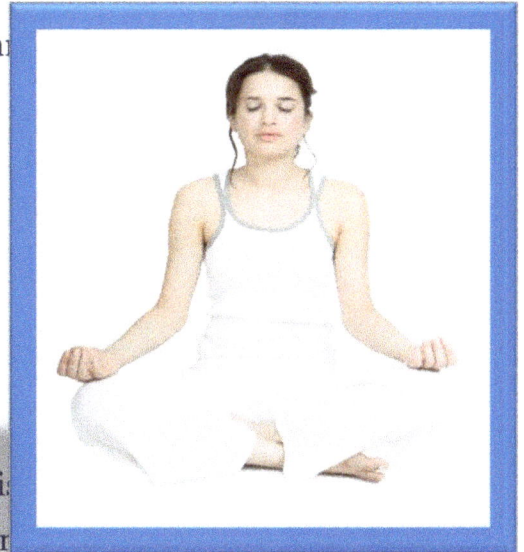

and hair growth in areas where there was no hair before! Many adolescents feel uneasy and uncomfortable about their bodies, including their feet!

Yoga and mindfulness are great forms of physical exercise for teens, helping them remain fit in any style they choose. Some teens may enjoy some gentle restorative yoga with others, and others may already be 'athletic' and opt for some Ashtanga. Either way, yoga is excellent for pumping the heart, moving the body, flowing blood, and twisting muscles, particularly after school days or lounging around their bedrooms being hunched over a desk or computer. In addition, keeping teenagers' active helps with weight loss, especially with the hormonal changes in their bodies that cause possible weight fluctuations.

Yoga is also excellent at building strength, although many asanas can build muscle and even bone strength when seen as a passive exercise! e.g., it is beneficial for budding dancers, gymnasts, and soccer players.

Yoga is especially significant because it helps stretch and warm up the body in a healthy way in preparation for high-energy exercise, so ideally, your 'sporty' kid will not come home with a broken knee, sciatic nerve, or back issues.

Yoga helps boost balance for 'academic' children who spend a lot of time hunched over chairs, screens, books, and heavy backpacks, which can avoid back problems later in life. Yoga facilitates the maintenance of an upright posture and strengthens the spine's back muscles and adjacent ones that support the spine.

Yogic breathing improves the lung ability, allowing the circulation and lymphatic systems to send more oxygenated blood through the body, thereby nourishing and cleaning every organ, muscle, nerve, and cell. According to Chinese medicine, blood stagnation can lead to discomfort (unease) in the body, leading to physical ailments later in life. Yogic breathing makes it possible for blood and oxygen to pass through the body, filtering away excess waste easily.

Relaxation Games for Kids

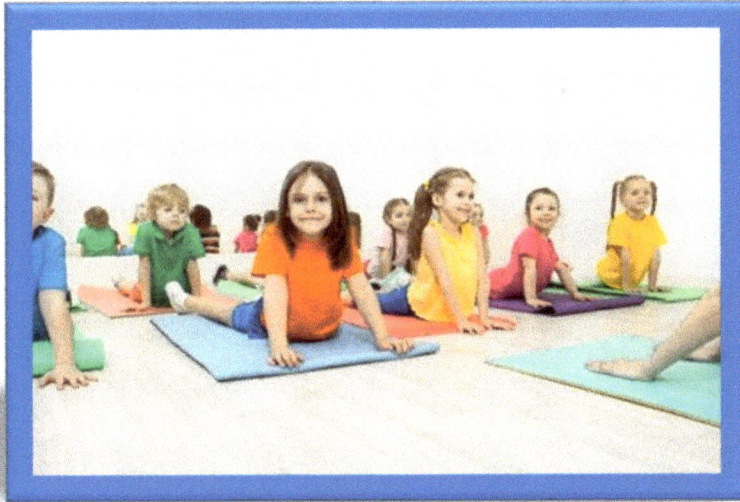

Games that help children use their imagination and think about things happening in their lives in the present can help them better understand what they should think about and make the most of their everyday surroundings.

Kids at home and school are displaying more and more mental health problems. Many teachers regard this situation as potentially negative for their physical and psychological wellbeing. Using relaxation games for children is an extraordinary idea, as it is visible to us that it makes them able to overcome their moods.

It is essential to pay attention to how your children's lives go by looking at how you lived at a young age. Children today live in a fast pace driven society; therefore, it would be wise for parents to provide their children with some good relaxation games to help them relax and think about the future when they are grown.

This will help create a harmonious atmosphere in the family. Anyone in the family can do this activity. This also helps strengthen the family's bond and makes for a strong relationship.

Advantages of relaxation for children

For an adult to relax, they have more natural ways to do so. For a child, a parent or a caregiver is more effective. For adults, a walk on the beach, a yoga class, or a conversation with friends is enough to release tension and heal the mind.

But for the little ones, video games form a great distraction away from all this emotional burden. Some of the advantages of this feature, when used for children or teenagers, are:

- Fights mental and muscle stress effectively.
- It helps to improve concentration and learning.
- It brings calm and peace.
- Reduces anxiety and panic attacks.
- When a state of relaxation is achieved, sleep improves.

Games to relax the family

1. Paint mandalas: This technique helps to relax children, youth, and adults. When painting a mandala, the brain's two hemispheres, the right, and the left, work together. To make this activity more enjoyable, it is possible to put soft music in the background. Many templates can be found on brochures, magazines, or the Internet. All we need to do is have the mandalas printed on paper so that everyone can colour them to taste. Otherwise, visit our website(www.newbeepublication.com) to buy activity books for adults and children.

2. Crumple, crush, and scribble papers: For this activity, you only need paper sheets placed on the table together with coloured pencils and pens to be scribbled at will. Subsequently, these sheets must be crushed until they form a ball, and then they must be crushed with the hands as if they were a ball of dough. In this way, each time the hands are opened and closed, the negative energies will be drained from the children, and they are fine motor skills will be developed.

The family, when playing together, shows support in these moments of tension. In this way, a calm environment is promoted to face any adversity with serenity and intelligence.

CHAPTER SEVEN
Meditation Exercises for Children

Children are bombarded today with excessive activities, screens, a lot of data... Their lives are busy, and little ones can experience stress, believe it or not, so kids' meditation exercises can help alleviate symptoms.

One of the parents' most typical ways to notice signs of stress, depression, or anxiety is to observe whether their child has trouble falling asleep. Other signs of stress in children include headaches, stomachaches, and hyperactivity. Thus, the solution may be meditation.

Meditation is a very efficient way of helping young people cope with stress and process it. In children, meditation can prevent stress and help heal those who face it.

It is also a great way to help little ones relax and unwind after a long day, preparing them for the sleep of a restful night.

To help your child get started, you do not need to have experience with meditation independently. So here are a couple of ways to start.

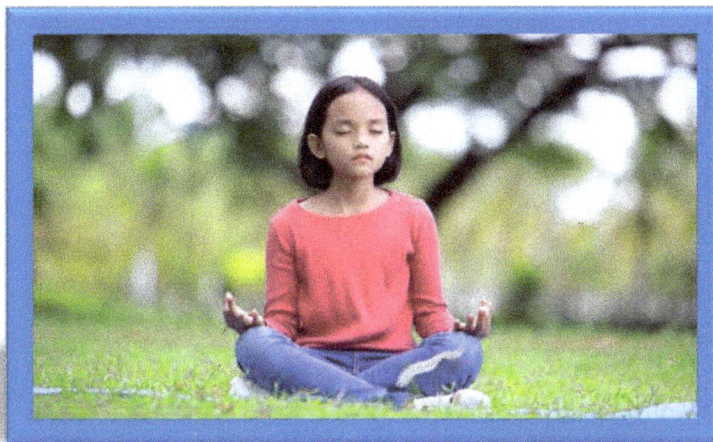

Meditation exercises for children

Meditation practices offer tools to calm their bodies, relax their minds, and help them cope with their thoughts.

Mindfulness meditations often focus primarily on the breath: children learn to turn their attention to the breath when their thoughts start to wander. This not only helps kids relax but also helps them focus better on school.

Code 6-2-7 can be an excellent way to start meditation.

Deep breathing

Deep breathing is a great technique to teach your child. Breathing is natural for us and helps us regulate ourselves in many ways. When a child becomes nervous, anxious, or stressed, deep breathing can help regain balance.

Teaching deep breathing at home can help him remember to use this technique during difficult times of the day.

When you have practised this technique for a while, you can make the sequences longer and longer and the breathing more profound. This technique is perfect for both adults and children who cannot fall asleep. Every time the mind wanders (which it will), it can refocus on counting and breathing.

Mantras in meditation

You can rehearse saying mantras with your child. In this sense, repeating the same prayer that both you and your child consider necessary can also help him meditate. Rehearse the sentence and adjust it so that it is easy to say; have your child repeat it with their eyes closed.

Some examples of mantras are:

- I love my life.

- I am always loved, and love comes easily to me.

- My heart is full of love, and I love myself more than anything.

- What does not suit me, I let go.

- I am thankful for.......

- I believe in myself

- I have total faith in my abilities

- I am ready for anything

- I know I can meet any challenges

- My body is healthy, and my mind is strong.

Meditation exercises for children at bedtime

Meditation exercises at bedtime are beneficial for calming the nervous system and reducing the child's stress hormones. In general, a child can meditate for the number of minutes equivalent to his age. However, if meditation makes your child relax, it can last longer and ease the transition to sleep.

To achieve this, you will have to provide a calm and peaceful environment in your child's bedroom, with soft lighting, soft music, and even aromatherapy. Your little one will learn to relax his mind and body, and it will be much easier for him to fall asleep and rest.

As you can see, there are different ways of meditation, and you can choose the one that best suits your children's needs and abilities.

Mindfulness and Meditation Activities for Families

Mindful meditation in individuals of all ages and cultures reduces anxiety, increases empathy, and promotes happiness and wellbeing.

It may seem like a stressful prospect to meditate with children, but this simple, ancient practice can take many forms and, in fact, be magnificent for little ones. Start with these easy and fun exercises to present the children with inner peace and to feel that the most stressful situations can be controlled within each family.

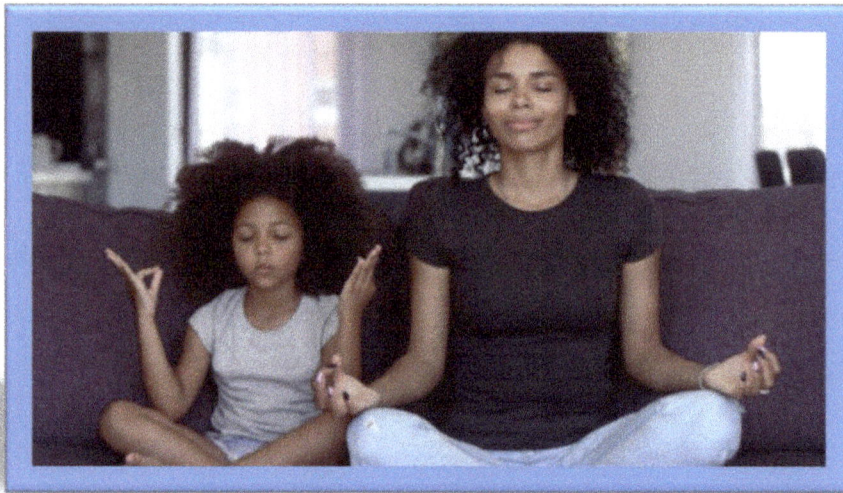

Family breathing: mindfulness and meditation

One of those biological reflexes that we do not even pay attention to is breathing. Yet, indeed it is something that we do well. So, an easy and instant way to inspire a few moments of quiet concentration is to learn how to take deep breaths to cleanse your body.

Ask your child to place his hands on his stomach and close his eyes. Encourage him, counting to five, to breathe deeply through his nose, hold his breath for two seconds and then count down as he exhales. Ask him to watch his tummy rise and fall as his lungs fill and the air is released.

Listening carefully

Mindfulness is about tuning in to the present moment without attachment or judgment and accepting it. Children are constantly moving both physically and mentally, coming and going between what happened at the end and what comes next. So, they still develop the gift of focusing on the here and now and enjoying it.

Challenge a game for your kids and ask them to sit with their legs crossed and their eyes closed. Then, ask them to listen carefully as you ring a bell, wind bell, or musical chords. Then, play a different kind of sound and ask them what sound that is.

After all, for each phase of life, patience and listening are essential abilities. Your children will learn to listen and be patient with this activity, something necessary for their personal and future professional lives.

Meditation and mindfulness before bed

Difficulties at bedtime make it difficult for night-time meditation, but ideal if you can integrate it into your routine. Guided meditation is done while lying, and relaxing the body is a good idea for the whole family, as it aims to calm the mind with relaxing instructions through audio.

You can ask your child to imagine, for instance, that he is a tree, to visualise his roots and branches, leaves, or flowers, as well as the field or forest where he is growing up and how he got there. Ask him to feel the sun's imaginary warmth and the earth's touch beneath him.

Speak slowly and include, between breaks, a long, exaggerated breath. Basically, before bed, this is the most relaxing story! "Before putting children to sleep, you can search YouTube for "sleep meditation for children" to find a relaxing host or ideas for your guided meditation routine.

Moving meditation

The kids love moving around. When trying to meditate with children, standing or sitting still can be a challenging factor. Make this a family activity, e.g., looking at the peaceful forest on YouTube example. You enjoy a time of family unity.

On top of a mountain, meditation is not just for monks. It is a fun and accessible activity that can be done anywhere by anyone. It may have a ripple effect of lifetime benefits to introduce this relaxing concept into children's lives from an early age.

CHAPTER EIGHT

Yoga in Schools

As a Yoga teacher, I have noticed that children get time for self-talk, self-care, and self-alignment during a yoga session, which helps them to stay calm and attentive for the whole day in school.

After trying yoga sessions in schools – the teachers noticed that the test scores increased more than 18% in less than two years, but the attendance rate decreased almost twice. The school has recorded that many students have reported that the school gets their participation up and feels them belonging.

Schools around the nation are introducing yoga in classrooms and beyond, with enormously positive results recorded by students, teachers, and parents.

Regulation of emotions

They need to develop self-regulation skills to excel in school and life: the ability to track and adjust their actions, attention, and emotions in response to internal indications, the environment, and others' input. And research indicates that the self-regulation of students can benefit from school-based yoga.

A randomised controlled study of 37 high school students, for example, found that doing 40 minutes of yoga three times a week for 16 weeks substantially enhanced their ability to control their emotions compared to taking part in a regular class in physical education (PE).

Furthermore, another study of 142 sixth graders compared students who practised four minutes of mindful yoga at the start of their English Language Arts (ELA) classes for a whole school year to students who received daily ELA classes, including a few brief discussions about mindfulness (but no mindful yoga). According to student questionnaires, the findings showed that this mindful yoga program often contributed to self-regulation improvements.

Academic performance

Most schools use academic achievement as the primary measure of student progress. Unfortunately, many learners struggle to attain or retain acceptable grades, leading them to drop out or disengage. But research indicates that yoga, three important factors for academic performance, could enhance concentration and memory and relieve academic stress.

School-based yoga could also enhance the grades of students. For example, one research randomly assigned 112 high school students to participate twice a week for 45 minutes during the entire academic year in either Yoga or PE. The yoga group ended up with a substantially higher grade point average (GPA) than the PE group among students with high participation levels.

95 high school students were allocated to participate in either a yoga program or a regular PE class by another similar randomised controlled study. The research found that students who participated in the yoga program could sustain their GPA, while during the 12-week program, students in the PE community saw a decrease in GPA.

"Yoga can enhance academic performance by improving self-regulation, which can, in turn, mitigate stress, leading to increased attention and learning," the authors write.

Reduced stress and anxiety

At school and home, children and teenagers are subject to several stressors. Such stressors may range from serious, persistent stress, such as poverty or violence, to relatively minor stressors, such as test anxiety. Adolescents with unmanaged stress are at increased risk of developing mental health conditions such as anxiety disorders, so some studies have researched whether school-based yoga can help relieve anxiety and stress.

Some students were assigned to engage in a mindful yoga program that met four days a week for 45 minutes in a randomised controlled trial of 97 fourth and fifth graders. As a result, 12 weeks of mindful yoga, compared to attending school as normal, led to substantial reductions in the problematic responses of students to stress, such as having repeated negative thoughts and intense, distracting emotions.

A Yoga 4 Classrooms program analysis showed a substantial decrease in cortisol concentrations from before to after the program for a group of 18-second graders who participated for half an hour per week for 10 weeks. During stress, cortisol in our saliva appears to increase, and elevated cortisol concentrations can be harmful to our mental and physical health due to repetitive stressors. This research offers tentative evidence that school-based yoga can help to reduce these adverse effects.

Stress resiliency

School-based yoga can also help students deal with adverse life events, such as home issues or bad grades in a significant class. A randomised controlled study of 155 fourth and fifth graders, for example, allocated several students to engage in a mindful eight-week yoga program that met for an hour a week. The study found that, relative to regular education, the yoga curriculum helped students deal with stressful life experiences more frequently.

Another research showed that 30 elementary and middle school students who participated once or twice a week in a 10-week yoga program strengthened their resilience-the ability to deal with stressful life events successfully.

Yoga practice increases the sense of control and self-efficacy concerning stress and emotion, thereby increasing resilience.

Less troublesome habits

Bullying happens very commonly in schools; over the past school year, about 28% of U.S. teenagers reported being harassed in 2011. Bullying can lead to a range of adverse effects on students, including academic achievement difficulties. Additionally, problem behaviours such as bullying also lead to suspensions and administrative referrals, meaning that they often miss valuable learning content.

But studies indicate that yoga might help. Third- to fifth-grade students, for example, who participated in a 10-week yoga program for one hour a week, showed less bullying after the program.

Similarly, another study allocated some of them to a semester-long, yoga-based social-emotional health program most days a week for half an hour for 159 sixth and ninth-grade students. Again, the findings showed that yoga community students had fewer absences and detentions without reason and were more interested in school compared to students who went to school as usual.

Such positive results may be attributed to yoga-based changes in understanding their emotions and actions by students. The researchers clarify that this could help students manage impulsive behaviours and negative responses to meet situational demands and achieve personal goals.

Well-being physical

According to the WHO - Worldwide obesity has nearly tripled since 1975. 38 million children under the age of 5 were overweight or obese in 2019, and over 340 million children and adolescents aged 5-19 were overweight or obese in 2016. A central factor at play is a lack of daily physical activity. Yoga is especially well- suited as a form of mindful movement to provide young people with non- competitive, gentle ways of participating in physical activity.

This 12-week study of 16 first-grade students who participated in 45 minutes of yoga twice a week showed that yoga, including balance, strength, and flexibility, can enhance motor skills. Furthermore, another study found that a year-long program of yoga-related exercises for 5-15 minutes per day improved students' physical wellbeing, including their body posture, sleep quality, exhaustion, and diet, based on surveys of hundreds of parents, students, and PE teachers.

"Yoga seems to be simply a stretching activity, but the variety and sequencing of postures coupled with deep breathing practice create an extremely diverse and effective way to improve a range of fitness abilities related to health."

Wellbeing for teachers and the environment in the classroom

Advocates for school-based mindfulness initiatives argue that these programs' benefits may influence the classroom environment and teachers' efficacy beyond students. Preliminary research on yoga programs for educators shows that yoga may also be beneficial for teachers' wellbeing.

Benefits of Classroom Meditation

Children do not feel as overwhelmed as adults by as many biases, obstacles, or preconceived ideas. When it comes to practising meditation, they, therefore, have an advantage.

First, we must keep in mind that meditation is an exercise both mentally and physically. Students who strive in the classroom and practice mindfulness enjoy its many short-and long-term advantages.

As part of regular teaching, meditation can play an important role. This allows students, as well as helping to see new perspectives, to increase their self-awareness.

The practice of meditation only requires dedication. After all, it is necessary to devote only 10 minutes a day and have a small space to sit comfortably.

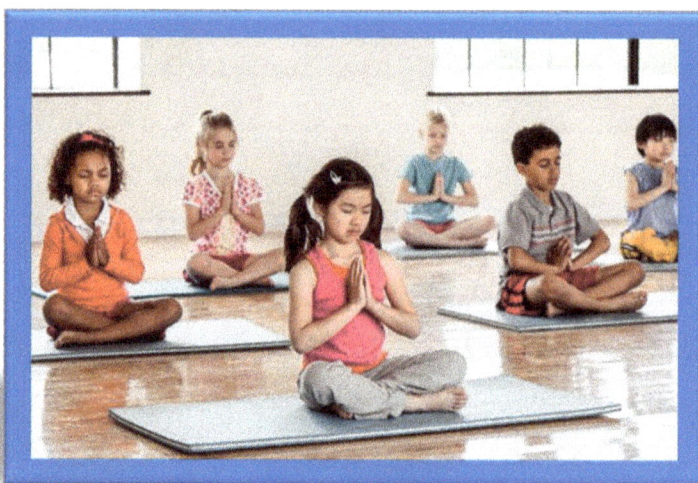

What are the benefits of classroom meditation?

1. Greater focus:

For more extended periods, meditation increases your capacity to concentrate. Likewise, it teaches children that their attention can be directed.

Students benefit from this in some ways, including paying attention for longer in class and thus, improving content retention.

2. Encourages compassion and self-esteem: Children sometimes feel that they will not pass an exam because of pressures and conditions beyond their control. This can be hard, particularly when others are scolding or mistreating you.

Luckily, meditation can reinforce the feelings of safety, empathy, and inner stability of children. When the whole class sits and does meditation together, it generates compassion, joy, and greater self-esteem.

3. Improves psychological wellbeing:

classroom meditation practice improves children's focus and decreases internalisation issues such as fear, non-integration into social groups, anxiety, and depression.

In this way, it improves their psychological wellbeing, as confirmed by several scientific studies.

4. Reduces stress:

Meditation provides children with the necessary time to rest physically, mentally, and emotionally, directly affecting the entire nervous system. This is because it reduces the production of chemicals related to stress, such as cortisol. Also, meditation lowers oxygen consumption, heart rate, respiratory rate, and blood pressure.

5. Improves memory:

This ability allows students to retain more information. This is essential to obtain better results in the tests and, thus, pass different tests.

Furthermore, a good memory means an increased ability to combine different ideas and thoughts simultaneously. So, this is a valuable skill for conducting intelligent and interesting conversations and reasoning.

6. Better control of emotions: Experts certify the relationship between emotional imbalance and negative results at school. Fortunately, as you may have noticed, one of the benefits of mindfulness is that it reduces stress and anxiety.

As if that were not enough, meditation also helps students better manage their emotions. Again, this has a positive impact on academic results.

In short, having time for students to relax mentally is essential to improving behaviour. Bearing in mind that children and young people are often in stressful situations, meditation is a way to get together and focus their thoughts.

Yoga schedule

Day	Time	Yoga poses	Practiced ✓

Day	Time	Yoga poses	Practiced ✓

REFERENCES

1. Exercise-benefits-cognitive-function-performance., (www.cnbc.com/2019/09/15/)

2. Neha Gothe, study author and director of the exercise psychology lab: The University of Illinois at Urbana-Champaign,

3. Sciencedirect.com

4. Addiction Rehab Toronto.

5. Kappmeier K. L., and D. M. Ambrosini. Instructing Hatha Yoga. Champaign, IL: Human Kinetics; 2006

6. Budilovsky, J., E. Adamson, and C. Flynn. The Complete Idiot's Guide to Yoga. 4th ed. New York, NY: Penguin Group; 2006

7. Kaminoff, L., and A. Matthews. Yoga Anatomy. 2nd ed. Champaign, IL: Human Kinetics; 2012

8. YogaJournal.http://www.yogajournal.com/poses/finder/browse_categories

9. Komitor, Jodi, and Eve Adamson.

10. The Complete Idiot's Guide to Yoga with Kids. Indianapolis, Indiana: Alpha Books, 2000.

If you like our book, please rate our effort by giving a review on Amazon.

OR

Visit our website for further publications

www.newbeepublication.com

www.ingramcontent.com/pod-product-compliance
Lightning Source LLC
Chambersburg PA
CBHW042350030426
42336CB00025B/3435